Women'sHealth

SHRINK YOUR SUGAR BELLY

ARE YOU
HOOKED
ON SUGAR?

PHOTOGRAPHY: JAMIE CHUNG

*Is your compulsion for sweets your biggest diet downfall? Find out
why sugar sabotages your weight loss– and how to fight back*

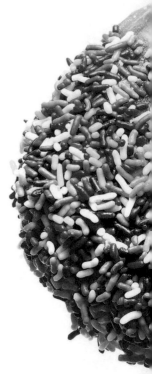

Before you say no, consider what you've put in your mouth lately. If it includes anything from breakfast cereal and coffee-shop beverages to cold cuts and ketchup, there's a decent chance you're riding a sugar rush right now. Don't feel bad – just about every person in the UK is buzzed. Research shows that nearly a quarter of our daily caloric intake – 512 calories on average – comes from sugar. But it is possible to free yourself from the diet-destroying confines of the sweet stuff. This book, brought to you by the experts at *Women's Health*, is here to show you how.

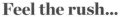

Feel the rush...

Sweet treats are bad news because they typically deliver a load of calories while offering little or no nutrition in exchange. And, more worryingly, as our consumption of the white stuff rises, so do the numbers on our scales.

What's really scary about sugar, though, isn't just its ability to make you put on more weight than you should. It's the way it *behaves*. Firstly, eating sugar often ends up stoking your appetite rather than satisfying it. And secondly, it can even become addictive – no surprise to those of us who have a daily 3pm chocolate craving that would tempt us to hurl an office chair at the vending machine if we ever ran out of change.

But there's no need for you to despair. There's light at the end of this frosted, icing-coated tunnel. With a little determination and some simple diet tweaks, you can train yourself to stop craving sugar. And when you do, you'll experience something truly sweet: successful, long-term weight loss.

Take your lumps

Even when you're fully aware that your favourite peanut butter is spiked with sugar, buying the unsweetened kind can feel like a major sacrifice. And that's just peanut butter – think of the croissant on the way to work; your co-workers' homemade biscuits; the caramel-flavoured cocktail in the sugar-rimmed glass at happy hour. There's a reason you keep coming back for more: you've got a habit.

In a study in *Physiology & Behavior*, a group of researchers found that eating sugar triggers the release of opioids, neurotransmitters that activate the brain's pleasure receptors. Addictive drugs, including morphine, target the same opioid receptors. "Sugar stimulates receptors to activate the same pathways that are stimulated directly by drugs such as heroin or morphine," the study reported.

So if you regularly swap your breakfast for a sweet coffee drink, you could be setting yourself up for sugar addiction that will influence the rest of your day's eating plans.

The replacements

How hooked you get on sugar may depend largely on what kind you eat. Fructose, the natural sugar found in fruit and certain vegetables, doesn't make you immediately feel as if you need another sugar hit, mainly because the fibre and other nutrients in those foods slow down the digestive process and help keep your blood-sugar level stable. That's one reason nutritionists always advise that you snack on fibre-rich fruit and not sweets.

But the main issue is that ever since the creation of that particular sugar, increasingly higher amounts of all sugars have found their ways into our diets – often in the least likely places. All that sugar can adversely affect the way we metabolise various foods.

And if getting too many calories is what worries you, reaching for a diet fizzy drink isn't the solution: artificial sweeteners may be almost as bad for you as common-or-garden sugar. A study published in the *International Journal of Obesity* found that rats ate more after consuming an artificially sweetened drink than they did after sipping sugar water.

Researchers speculate that calorie-free artificial sweeteners act like stomach teasers: as you swallow diet drinks, your body anticipates the arrival of calories. When they don't show up, your body sends you looking elsewhere for them.

A study by researchers from the University of Texas found that people who drank a can of a diet drink every day had 37 per cent greater incidence of obesity. And because artificial sweeteners are often many times sweeter than sugar, stirring a teaspoonful into your daily cup of Java may mean that when you do use real sugar, it just doesn't taste sweet enough for you, sending you grabbing for extra sugar packets.

Cut the sugar, shrink your belly

Here comes the hard-to-swallow truth: the only way to curb a sugar habit is to cut back drastically. It will be rough in the beginning, but your body will crave sugar less as it regains its insulin sensitivity. In order to extract your sweet tooth, you first need to know how much sugar you're actually eating.

There are plenty of hidden sources of sugar and a wide range of sweeteners – learn their names and you'll dodge their attempts to sneak into your diet. Read labels on the foods that you're eating for a week and keep an eye on how much sugar, on average, you're taking in – the NHS recommends a limit of 10 per cent of your daily caloric intake, which is about 50 grams, or 10 teaspoons.

You'll also realise that many products that are touted as healthy are still high in sugar. There are no laws regulating the use of the words "all natural" on food packaging, so manufacturers can label their products with abandon. One ounce of dried pineapple has about 21 grams of sugar, compared with 2.6 grams for the same amount of fresh pineapple. So watch your portions.

The first few days of your *Sugar Belly Shrink* plan will involve this kind of monitoring and analysis of exactly what's going into your shopping basket and your mouth. We believe that it's the best way of fending off the sugars that sneak into your diet – and securing room for the sugars that you'll choose to treat yourself with once the plan is completed.

TAKE YOUR LICKS
Could your tastebuds be 'sugar blind'?

Scientific research has found that we all have a different number of taste buds on our tongues. The amount you have puts you into one of three groups: non-tasters, who, on average, have five taste buds in an area the size of a paper hole punch; supertasters, who have about 30; and medium tasters, who fall in between. The non-tasters need lots of sugar to taste sweetness; supertasters are satisfied with a tiny bit. This is why a piece of chocolate cake can seem too rich.

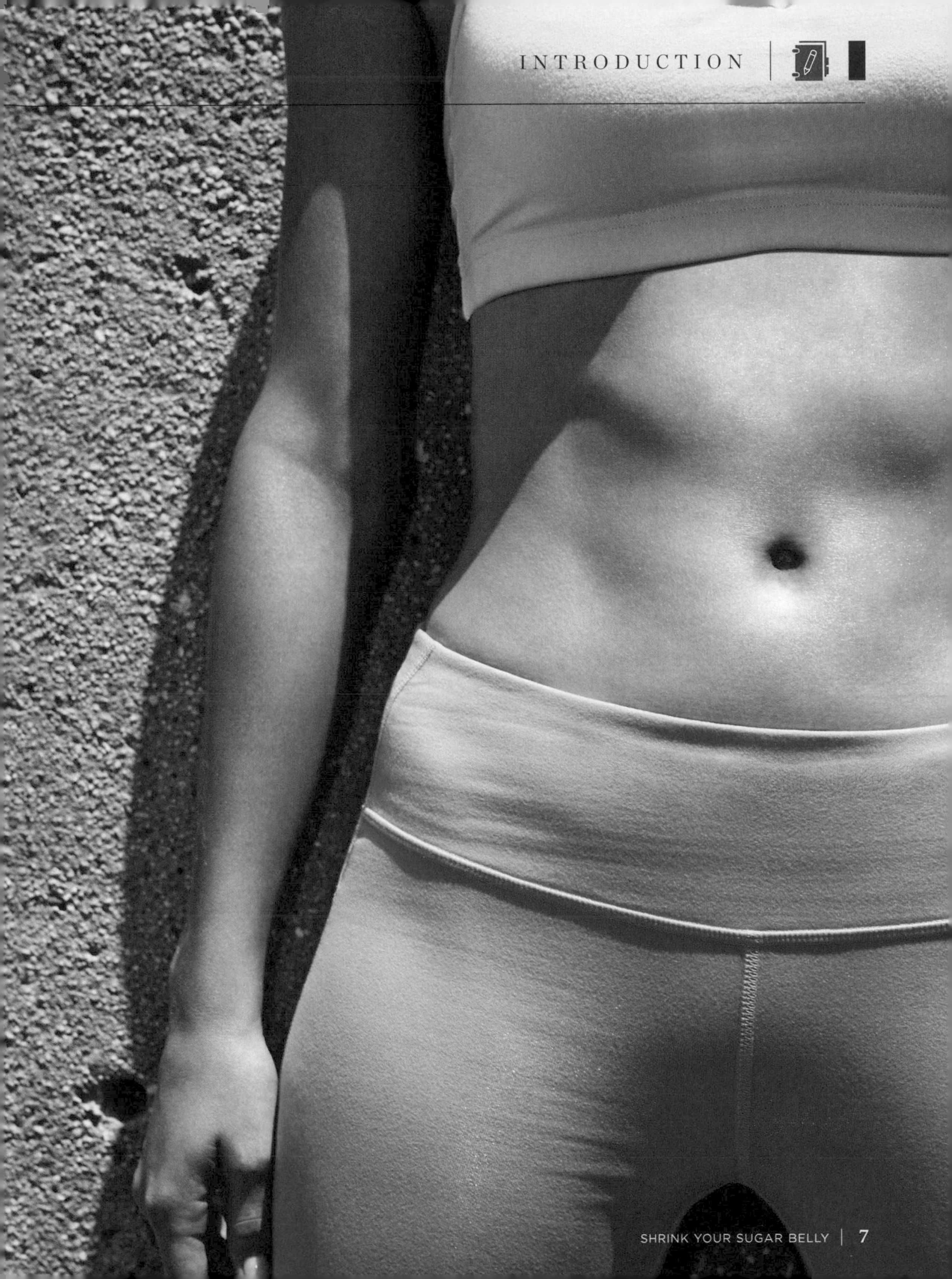

CONTENTS

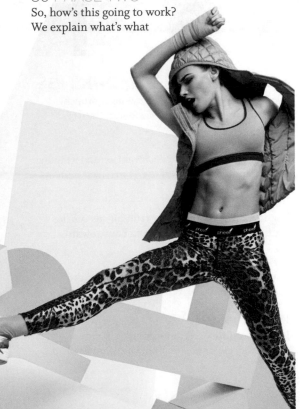

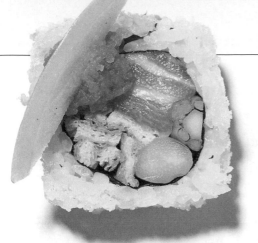

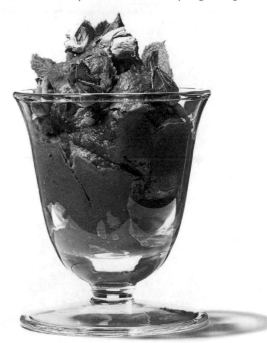

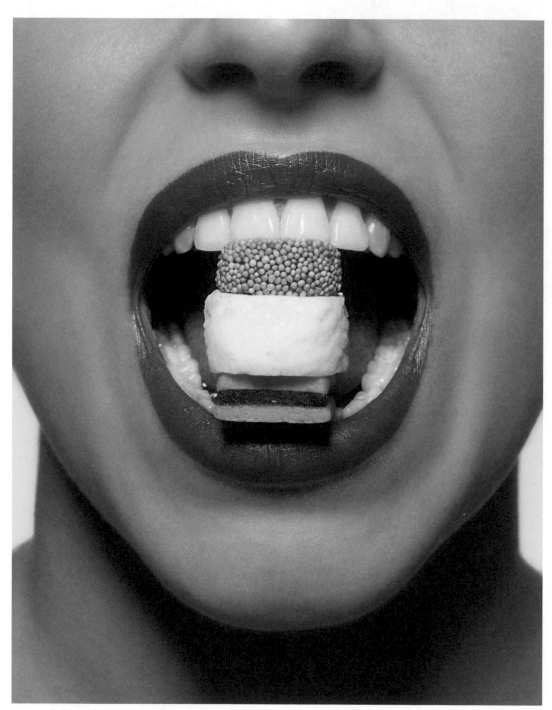

ALL ABOUT SUGAR

✦ THE SCIENCE ✦ THE PLAN ✦ THE RULES ✦

The biggest changes always happen when you first understand how – and why – these decisions will benefit you. Before you start your 20 days of sugar-belly shrinkage, let's talk about the unique impact sugar makes on your body, and the far-reaching benefits to your health, waistline and complexion when you start to shun it

14 The Sugar-Belly Connection
What is this extra padding round your waist, and why won't it go away? When you learn how your body stores and reacts to sugar, you'll want to change the way you eat forever.

24 Introducing the Eating Plan
There's a 20-day journey ahead of you, some of it hard going while your brain and body ditch their sugary habits. Find out what to expect on the way there, and the prize that awaits you at the end.

36 Eight Rules for Success
The meals are delicious, but chances are your body will still cry out for its sugar fix. Let us be your guide: follow these simple principles to minimise cravings and quieten a busy mind.

THE
SUGAR-BELLY
CONNECTION

Found in the most innocent-looking food, sugar is enemy number one. Now it's time to re-educate your taste buds

We all know that cutting sugar from our diet is good for our health and waistline, but how many of us know why? The answer lies in the difference between the fat on your belly and what's stored on the rest of your body. The non-belly fat – the pinchable stuff on our thighs and backsides – is called subcutaneous fat. It's actually pretty friendly in healthy doses, acting as a storage depot for energy. But belly fat is a different matter. It's actually active, so much so that it's now regarded as an organ in its own right. It churns out nasty substances that impair healthy body function – and it likes to add to itself. We refer to this lurking nasty as the 'sugar belly'.

How does belly fat develop? It all begins with your body's ability to balance two substances: glucose and insulin. Your muscles and brain rely on glucose for energy, and insulin is a hormone released by your pancreas to help move that glucose from your bloodstream into the muscle and brain cells that use it. The more glucose in your blood, the more insulin

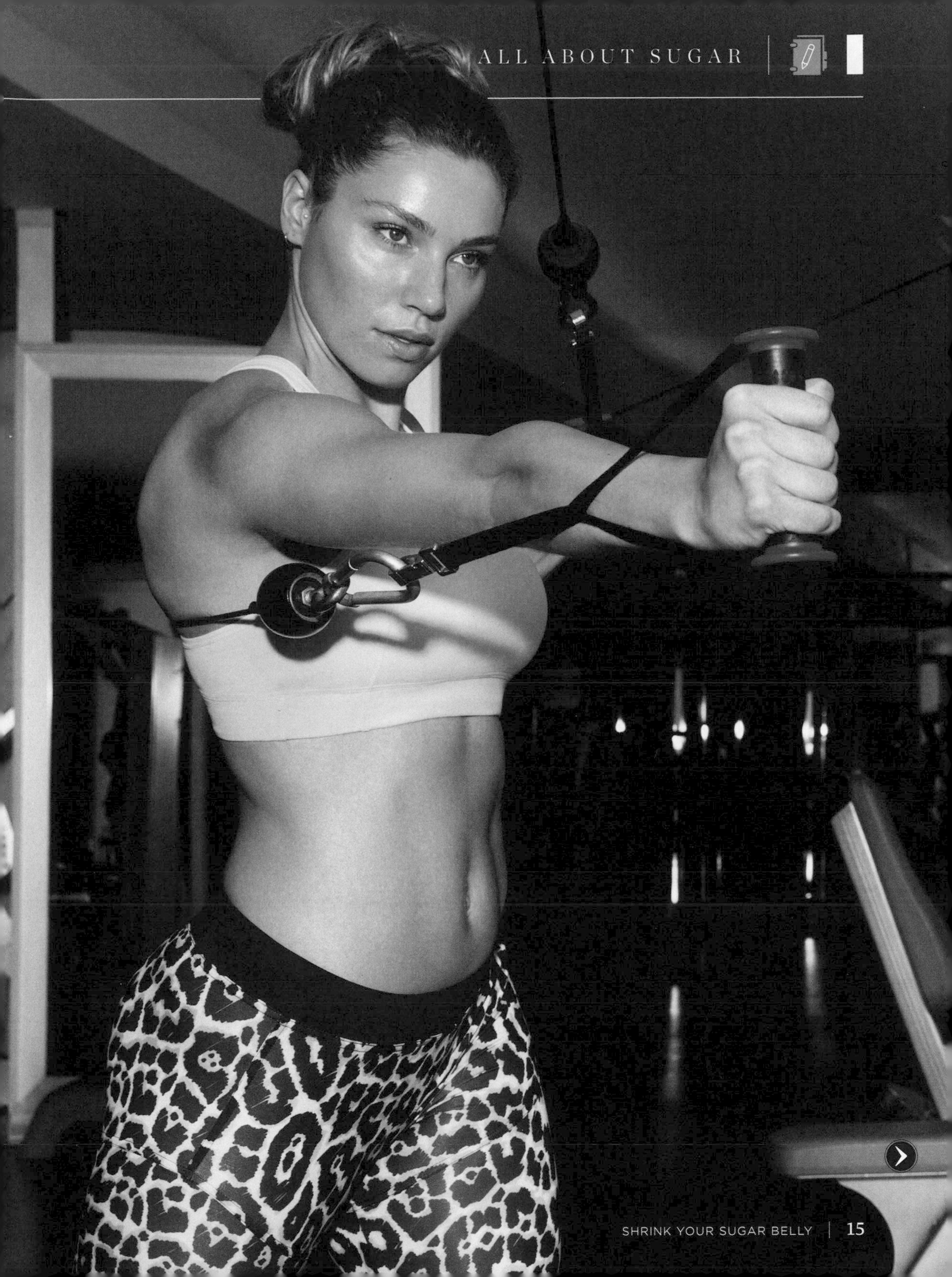

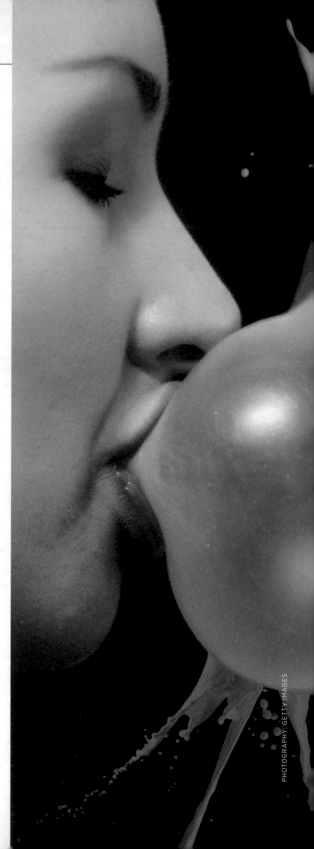

your body needs. And that's in this simple chemical relationship that sugar belly problems start.

During digestion, your body breaks down food into its individual components: amino acids (from protein), fatty acids (from fat) and glucose (from carbohydrates). When your body takes in quickly-digested carbohydrates, your bloodstream becomes quickly flooded with a large amount of glucose – resulting in the production of a corresponding quantity of insulin in order to transport it.

Which carbs are digested quickly? Sugar is one of the speediest. But so are refined carbohydrates like white flour, as well as many processed wholegrain products. For instance, the kind of wholewheat bread typically used for sandwiches and white bread are digested at

We are designed to handle fructose in small amounts, not the 49kg of sugar a year the average Brit consumes

about the same rate and cause about the same rise in blood glucose levels, and therefore require the same amount of insulin to clear the bloodstream of glucose.

Over time, repeated, extreme spikes in insulin have several detrimental effects on your body's ability to correctly digest and store food. First, your cells become less responsive to it. This condition, insulin resistance, results in your pancreas producing even more insulin to compensate.

Glucose levels stay high, and in large amounts glucose can damage blood vessels and nerves. On top of that – and here's the link to your sugar belly – all that extra insulin floating around causes your body to store more fat than it normally would. It also prevents your body from using fat for energy between meals, and once it enters, it's not coming out. Think of it as a tattoo – easy to get on your body in moments of abandon, and bloody hard to get off.

Think this is bad? You haven't heard the worst of it. Because your body is held back from using your stored fat for fuel, you become more hungry, more often. Then you produce more insulin and you store more fat. The more fat you have, the more resistant your cells become to insulin. It's a vicious cycle!

And this brings us to sugar – the cherry on the whole miserable cake. Insulin resistance promotes fat storage everywhere on your body. It's fructose, on the other hand, that contributes to belly fat specifically, according to studies. It's found naturally in fruits and some vegetables that are packaged with vitamins, minerals, phytochemicals and fibre. Not that fruit salad is the problem.

The real issue is that the amounts of fructose we're consuming in added sugars, such as table sugar (cane or white sugar), are swelling our bellies and menacing our health. Our bodies were designed to handle fructose in small amounts (ie: in a few servings of fruit or a little honey a day), not the 49kg of sugar a year the average Brit consumes. And in this form, you aren't getting any of the good stuff – like fibre or vitamins – along with it.

Don't assume heart disease and diabetes are years away; too much fructose takes a toll on even young hearts, according to a study published in the *Journal of Nutrition*. It found that teens who consumed the most fructose had higher blood pressure and blood-sugar levels than those who ate the least, and it linked high-fructose diets to increases in visceral fat.

FROM SUGAR BELLY TO FATTY LIVER

Located on the right side of your abdomen, tucked behind your lower ribs, lies your liver – the body's alchemist. One of its most critical jobs is to turn toxins – both formed naturally in the body and man-made, such as medication and alcohol – into harmless substances. This hardworking organ uses about 20 per cent of the calories you take in to fuel itself and its critical work, which also includes converting proteins and sugars from food into energy for your body.

Recent research suggests that calories from different types of food are metabolised differently in the body. Every single one of your body's 10 trillion cells can metabolise glucose. But only the liver can

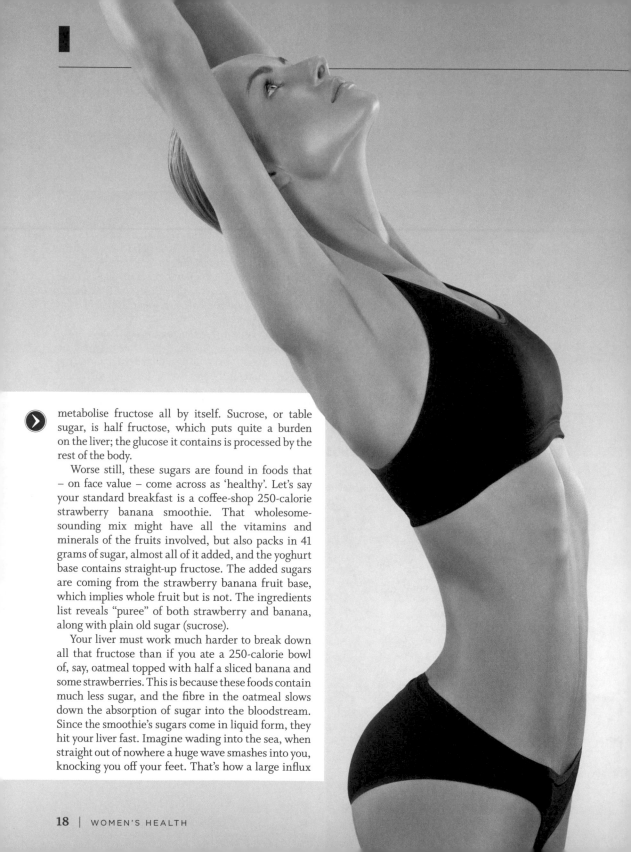

metabolise fructose all by itself. Sucrose, or table sugar, is half fructose, which puts quite a burden on the liver; the glucose it contains is processed by the rest of the body.

Worse still, these sugars are found in foods that – on face value – come across as 'healthy'. Let's say your standard breakfast is a coffee-shop 250-calorie strawberry banana smoothie. That wholesome-sounding mix might have all the vitamins and minerals of the fruits involved, but also packs in 41 grams of sugar, almost all of it added, and the yoghurt base contains straight-up fructose. The added sugars are coming from the strawberry banana fruit base, which implies whole fruit but is not. The ingredients list reveals "puree" of both strawberry and banana, along with plain old sugar (sucrose).

Your liver must work much harder to break down all that fructose than if you ate a 250-calorie bowl of, say, oatmeal topped with half a sliced banana and some strawberries. This is because these foods contain much less sugar, and the fibre in the oatmeal slows down the absorption of sugar into the bloodstream. Since the smoothie's sugars come in liquid form, they hit your liver fast. Imagine wading into the sea, when straight out of nowhere a huge wave smashes into you, knocking you off your feet. That's how a large influx

insulin. As the pancreas churns out more and more of this fat-storage hormone to prod the liver into doing its job, insulin levels increase – and so does body fat.

FRUCTOSE: THE QUICKER FATTER-UPPER

As you'll recall, one of the liver's jobs is to convert the sugars in food into fuel for the body. It's also tasked with turning excess energy into body fat. This process is called lipogenesis, and, at least theoretically, research suggests the body may turn fructose into body fat more efficiently compared to sucrose and glucose.

An early study that looked for a link between fructose consumption and body fat was conducted on mice. German researchers allowed them to freely drink plain water or fructose-sweetened water – the rodent version of soft drinks – for 10 weeks. Though the fructose-sipping mice regularly ate fewer calories from solid food, they gained weight and ended up with 27 per cent more body fat than the mice that drank plain water. Because fructose doesn't need insulin to enter the cells, it floods the body and is quickly stored as fat.

Another study, this one on people, addressed the question of whether fructose really does cause the body to pack on fat. Researchers at the University of Texas Southwestern Medical Center fed 'breakfast' to six volunteers – four men and two women. The breakfast was actually lemonade that contained three different combinations of sugar – 100 per cent glucose, an equal mix of glucose and fructose, and 25 per cent glucose and 75 per cent fructose.

Immediately afterwards, the team measured the conversion of the sugars to fat in the liver. Four hours later, the volunteers ate lunch – turkey sandwiches, salty snacks and biscuits. Each volunteer's lunch contained different amounts of sugars based on body weight. Then the researchers measured how the food was metabolised. The results: lipogenesis rose 17 per cent when the volunteers had the fructose-containing drinks, compared to eight per cent for

---

of fructose hits your liver.

Keep cramming enough fructose in for long enough and globules of fat will begin to form in the cells of your liver. Before 1980, doctors rarely saw this fatty buildup, known as nonalcoholic fatty liver disease (NAFLD). Now, it affects one in five of all adults in the UK. It's worth noting that the rise in NAFLD has happened at exactly the same time as the increase in obesity, and that the condition affects between 70-90 per cent of people whose weight is graded at that level. In fact, experts consider NAFLD a hallmark of a condition characterised by the cluster of obesity

> **Cirrhosis only happens with really severe alcoholism, right? Now, it appears, an excessively sugary diet could play a role too**

related conditions known as metabolic syndrome.

This fat buildup in the liver isn't obvious on your body, either. An *American Journal of Clinical Nutrition* study found that people who ate 1,000 extra calories of sugary foods for three weeks saw just a two per cent increase in body weight, but a 27 per cent increase in liver fat.

When you lose weight, liver fat returns to normal levels. But if NAFLD isn't caught in time, the liver can become inflamed, which can lead to a more severe liver condition known as nonalcoholic steatohepatitis. If the inflammation becomes severe, scar tissue replaces healthy tissue, impairing the liver's ability to perform its crucial functions. When that happens, it's called cirrhosis. (Cirrhosis only happens with really severe alcoholism, right? Now, it appears, an excessively sugary diet could play a role, too.) A fat-riddled liver may become resistant to the action of

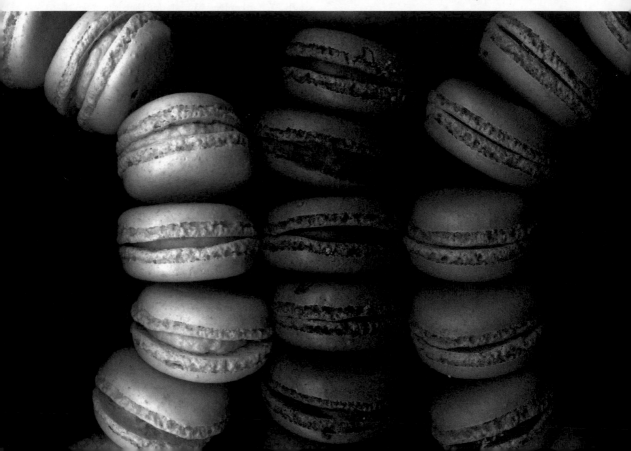

the glucose drink. Simply put, their bodies made fat more efficiently. Further, after metabolising fructose in the morning, the liver increased the storage of fats eaten at lunch. As the study's lead researcher, Dr Elizabeth Parks, put it: "The carbohydrates came into the body as sugars. The liver took the molecules apart and put them back together to build fats. All this happened within four hours of the fructose drink. As a result, when the next meal was eaten, lunch fat was more likely to be stored than burned." Although this research is preliminary, it raises questions about starting your day with a fructose-filled sugary drink.

Most likely, these results underestimated the effect of fructose because the test subjects were healthy and lean, and could process the fructose quickly. So the fat-packing potential of fructose may be worse if you're overweight, because this process is already revved up.

YOUR BRAIN, ON DOUGHNUTS

There's evidence that a steady diet of sugary, processed foods can mess with insulin in our brains, triggering what some experts are calling type-3 diabetes, better known as Alzheimer's disease. Researchers at Brown University in Rhode Island, USA, uncovered the link between insulin resistance and a high-fat diet in brain cells.

In a paper published in *Current Alzheimer Research*, they reviewed evidence suggesting that Alzheimer's is a metabolic disease in which the brain's ability to use glucose and produce energy is impaired. The evidence, they concluded, suggests that Alzheimer's has "virtually all of the features of diabetes, but is largely confined to the brain". In one study, they interfered with the way rats' brains naturally respond to insulin. The rats went on to develop all the brain damage seen in Alzheimer's, and were unable to learn their way through the kind of maze they normally had no problem navigating.

People with type-2 diabetes have been found to be significantly more likely to suffer from Alzheimer's. While the disease doesn't necessarily cause Alzheimer's, both diseases may share the same root: insulin resistance.

YOUR STONE-AGE SWEET TOOTH

So, why do our brains want more sugar than our bodies can handle? It sometimes seems as though Mother Nature has left us with a ticking time-bomb compulsion to self-destruct in the tastiest way possible, when you think how easy it is to lay your hands on the stuff. The answer lies back in the beginnings of our species – unsurprisingly in an era before corner shops.

It's thought that our ancestors associated a sweet taste with energy-dense, immune-system-protecting fruit. With survival of the entire human race hingeing on getting enough to eat, every calorie literally represented a matter of life and death, and a sweet taste triggered a reassuring 'this is safe to eat' message in ancient brains.

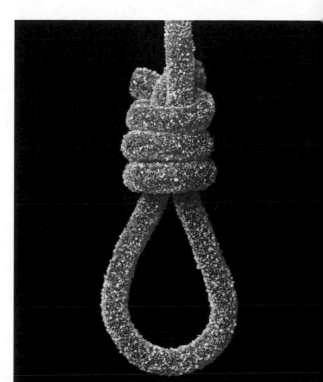

> **Our bodies were designed to crave a sugar that is supposedly hard to come by; store it quickly, and use it fast**

For a while, calorie-dense fruit and honey were virtually all we knew of sweet tastes. In the Paleolithic era (a period of half a million years that ended 10,000 years ago), fruits and vegetables made up well over half of our diet. But everything changed with the dawn of farming. As humans began to rely on cereal grains, our consumption of fruit and vegetables dropped. And sugar – derived from sugar cane, which was grown in tiny amounts at first – began

its relentless seduction of our taste buds. Our bodies were designed to crave a sugar that is supposedly hard to come by; store it quickly, and use it fast.

Our sugar-belly problem comes from when we're living in high-tech times – where one can access countless spoonfuls of the stuff in a single lunchtime – but still have brains that are hardwired to seek sugar. We simply end up storing more than we use. We're not climbing trees to pluck precious, high-hanging fruit; we're calling up for free delivery.

This is where the *Shrink Your Sugar Belly* eating plan comes in, cleverly exploiting your body's natural attraction to sugar while still allowing its healthy nutritional needs to be fulfilled. As you'll find, something as simple as the daily consumption of a protein-packed breakfast helps rein in your appetite during the day and reduces your urge to snack.

PHOTOGRAPHY: GETTY IMAGES

SHRINK YOUR SUGAR BELLY | 21

THE EMOTIONAL CONNECTION

We love sweet. Our taste buds, our eyes, our emotions – they all crave the reward of sugar. We love the taste, the way it makes us feel and the connection that sweet provides. Horrendous day? Ice cream. Crushing worries about your love life? Ice cream. Feeling fat and friendless? You get the idea. Eating in response to emotions like boredom, loneliness or anxiety – what's called emotional eating – is real.

In fact, in a study of 40 women of varying sizes, those who scored higher on a scientifically designed food-addiction scale showed more activity in the parts of the brain associated with addiction when they were shown a tempting image of a milkshake. One sign of using sugar to manage emotions is that responding to sugar craving doesn't alleviate it. Trying to satisfy the craving only prompts a desire for more... and more.

Habit ties us into an emotional attraction, too. If you're used to having a muffin for breakfast, biscuits in the afternoon or dessert after dinner, something starts to feel wrong if you skip it.

WHERE'S YOUR SUGAR LURKING?

We all know to steer clear of fizzy drinks because of their obvious sugar content. But you wouldn't have that same trepidation over a turkey sandwich on wholewheat bread – despite the fact that the bread alone can have up to two teaspoons of added sugar per slice. (If you want to continue shrinking your sugar belly after the eating plan you should be consuming no more than nine teaspoons of added sugar a day.) It's one thing to knowingly consume a sugar bomb. It's another to learn that many foods you consider healthy can be sugar bombs, too. Ultimately, there are two types of sugars in food: the kind you know about and the kind you don't.

Something as simple as breakfast, and packing it with protein, reins in your appetite

STRAIGHT-UP SUGAR Found in sweets, drinks, breakfast cereals, energy bars and desserts, this type of sugar is loud and proud. While it's often listed as 'sugar', it might also be called by different names. Even if you're aware that these foods pack sugar, you may not realise just how much. For instance, doesn't a chilled fruit drink sound better than Coke? A 500ml bottle of Coke has just over 13 teaspoons of sugar. A 500ml

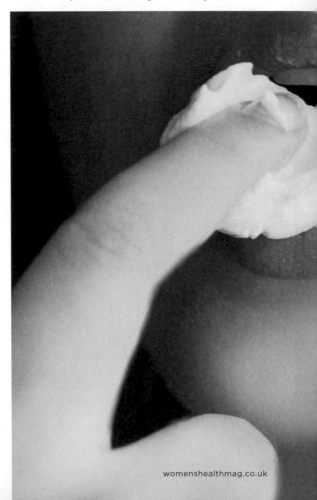

Oasis Summer Fruits has just over nine – better, but not by much. If you're following the sugar-belly-shrinking limits, that's your whole day's allowance in one bottle!

SECRET SUGAR Wander around your supermarket. Pick up bottles, jars and boxes at random and look at the ingredients lists. There will be a list of values titled 'of which sugars'. But more often than not, you're likely to find sugar listed as an ingredient, even if you don't recognise its alias. True to their name, Secret Sugars lurk in foods you don't even think as sweet. These include pasta sauce, packet noodles, salad dressings, ketchup, barbecue sauce and some deli meats and sausages. There are also sweeteners that you may not realise are sugar. It's frustrating, but once you're familiar with the many words for sugar in an ingredients list, you'll be better prepared to control your sugar choices.

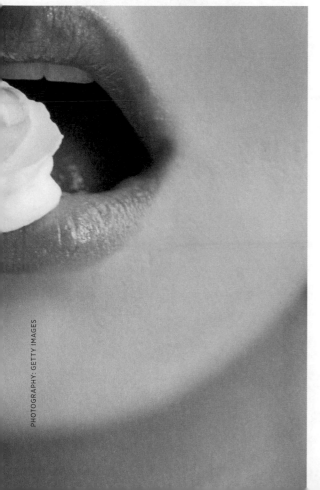

PHOTOGRAPHY: GETTY IMAGES

SUGAR MIMICS This is sugar in its sneakiest form: foods that don't taste like sugar but mimic its action in the body. Foods like crisps, bagels, potatoes, white rice and pasta may not contain sugar *per se*, but they might as well – they're digested as rapidly as sugar. And they have the same effect on the body: glucose floods the bloodstream, triggering a rise in the fat-storage hormone insulin and disruptions in other hormones that keep your appetite under control. So, as you'll be finding out, Sugar Mimics have the same harmful effects as Straight-Up and Secret Sugars.

You may know that a steady diet of refined carbohydrates, stripped of their fibre and nutrients, is associated with obesity and disease. Not your problem? You start the day with wholewheat toast or bran cereal. You snack on wholegrain crackers and hummus. Occasionally, you splurge on a wholegrain bagel. Wholegrain is healthy. Right? Not quite. If your wholegrain intake consists of foods made with wholegrain flour, like some cereals and crackers, you can also grow a sugar belly.

In the process of making wholewheat or wholegrain flour, kernels are pulverised practically to dust, so they're digested by your body about as quickly as white flour or table sugar. This means they can spike your blood sugar and insulin levels, leading to hunger and prompting you to reach for more of these foods. You're caught in an unending cycle of cravings and consumption.

But that cycle can be broken, and this book can help you do it. Everything you've read in these last few pages is pretty depressing, but the good news is that the solution lies in the delicious, filling recipes, simple workouts and smart tips to be found in the rest of this book. Isn't it time to get off the sugar merry-go-round and quench those formidable cravings once and for all? In the next chapter you'll learn how to hit 'Factory Reset' on your taste buds over just 20 days. But before that, let's find out exactly what's to come....

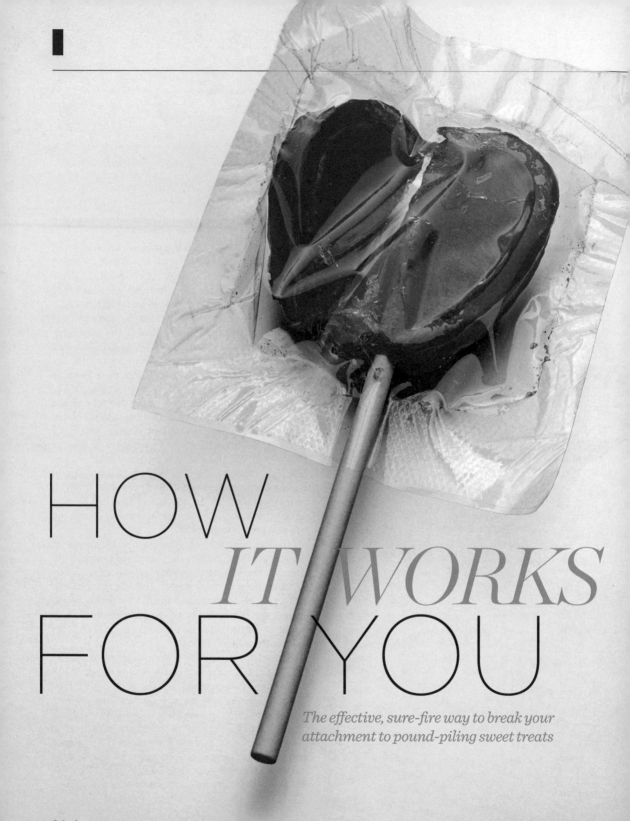

HOW *IT WORKS* FOR YOU

The effective, sure-fire way to break your attachment to pound-piling sweet treats

How will we get you to this point, where you're no longer enslaved by sugar and wobble-free at your waist? The *Shrink Your Sugar Belly* 20-day plan's success relies on a combination of eating whole, natural foods, physical activity, emotional-coping strategies and other tips to outsmart sugar cravings without feeling hungry or deprived. It gradually weans you off both obvious and hidden sugars and refined carbs so you can reintroduce sugar in a healthy, balanced way.

How do we define success? Of course, you'll see changes in your weight and measurements. But the side effects of your slimmer midriff should be just as pleasing – more energy, better sleep, clearer skin and fewer cravings. This plan is designed to help you redefine your relationship with sugar, not banish it from your life. Take a look at what's ahead, and you'll see that it offers everything you need to make that peace: self-awareness, knowledge, ways to apply that knowledge to everyday life, and – above all – choices.

Days 1–5

Your vital preparation days, where you'll use the resources in Chapter 2 to assess your intake of sugar (in all its forms) and refined grains, and gradually eliminate them. In just 72 hours, you'll begin to transform your physiological and emotional connection and reduce the effects of sugar overload.

Days 6–12

These are the tough-love days. Tough, because this phase removes sugar – even from fruit – from your diet. Love, in that you'll love the results: you should have lost an average of four pounds by Day 12. You also won't be eating any processed grain products, refined or wholegrain. Believe us, this will be an adjustment, but your dedication will chip away at sugar withdrawal and replace the temporary reward of a sugar rush with healthier routes to pleasure.

Days 12–20

It's time to get fruity. Nature's treat is back – in healthy amounts. You'll be amazed at how satisfying it will taste now that you've reset your taste buds. Low-sugar, wholegrain bread products return, too.

Day 21... and beyond!

From here on, it's up to you. Once you've learned to really think about the sugars you need in your life – and the ones you don't – you can enjoy the delicious meals, snacks, smoothies and desserts in the rest of the book. You'll discover the sugar substitutes that work and the low-sugar versions of treats that you already love. All of these meals will keep you full, give you energy and nourish your hair and skin, as well as whittling away your waist.

The sugar-belly burners

Enjoy these workouts as often as you can during your eating plan – and after! The more muscle you have, the better equipped your body is to process sugar and carbs. Exercise also helps boost mood and control belly-expanding stress. And it burns calories and fat.

That's just 20 days to a more healthy relationship with sugar. Prepare to enjoy one of life's greatest treats on your own terms, in ways that enhance your health and wellbeing without skimping on pleasure. Get ready to live the real sweet life...

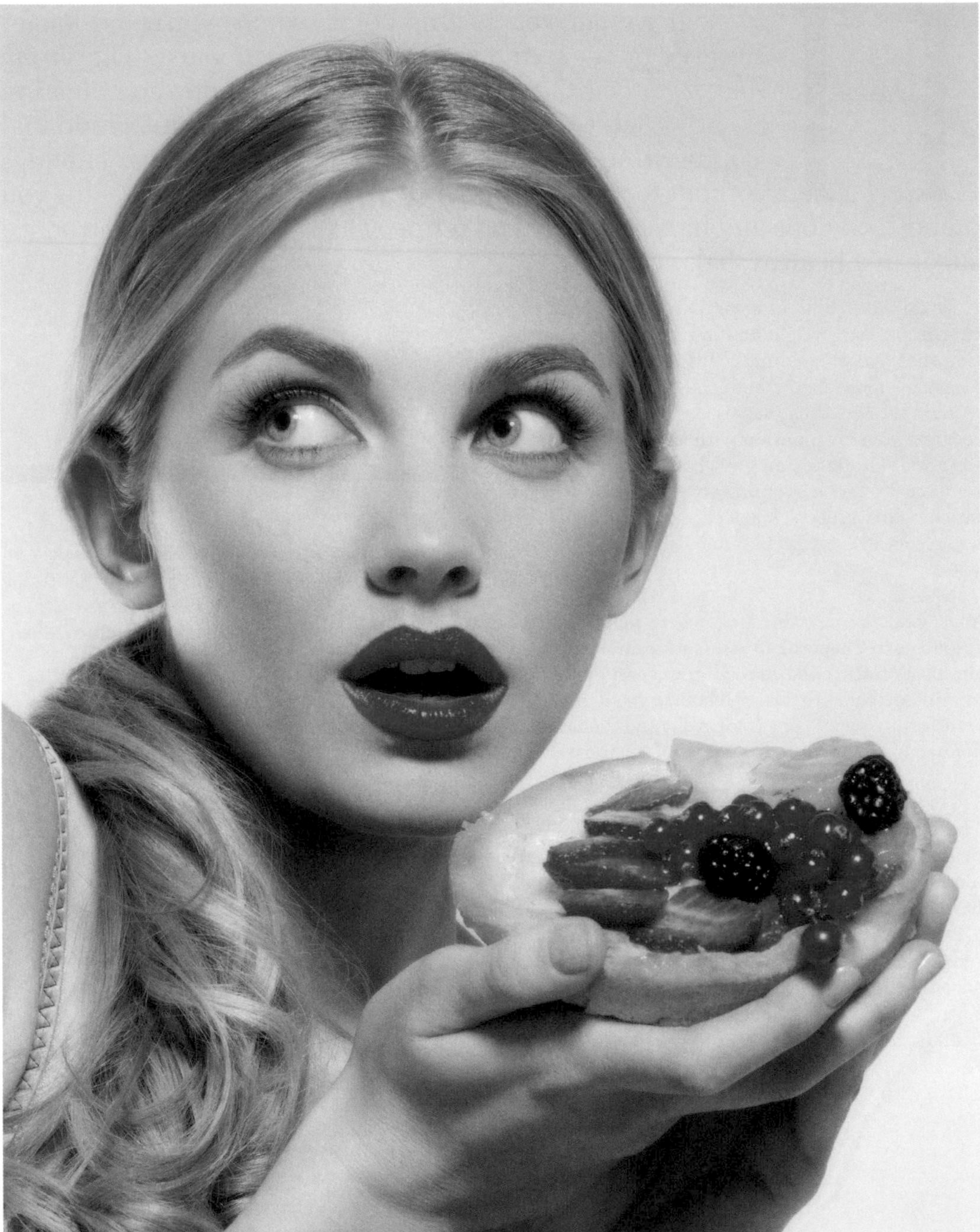

PHOTOGRAPHY: GETTY IMAGES

DAYS 1-5

+ PAUSE + ANALYSE + PREPARE + SUCCEED! +

Welcome to Day 1. You could cut all sugar from here on – forever! – but do you really think that will work? Let's face it, the white stuff isn't just a foodstuff you can pick up and put down. It's a reward, a celebration, a pick-me-up – and sometimes a friend. Boost your chances of success by preparing your mind and body (and fridge) first.

28 The Step Down
The *Women's Health* experts explain why self-awareness is essential for sugar-shunning success.

30 Day 1-2
Uncover your emotional links to sugar – and use your new knowledge against it!

38 Day 3
Learn to spot the Straight-Up Sugars lurking in your kitchen – and start making them disappear.

42 Day 4
Spot the sneakier sugars in your diet, and learn how to break the habits of sugar consumption.

46 Day 5
Get shopping for the first stage of the eating plan and create your 'personal-rewards card'.

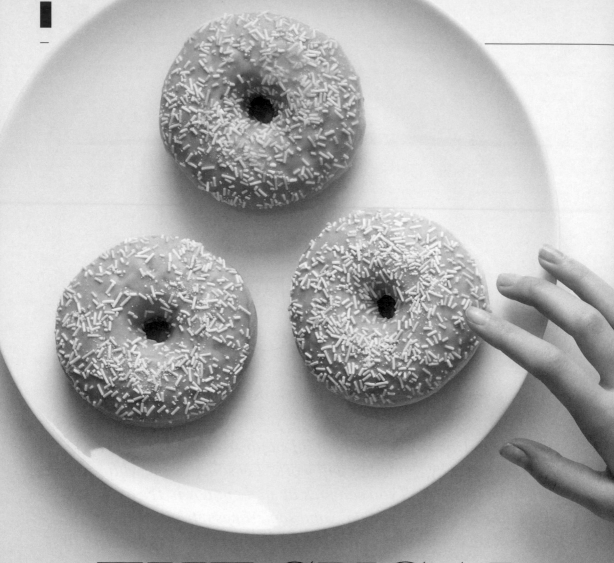

THE SUGAR STEP-DOWN

You're probably aware that you're not the only person with a 'close' relationship to sugar, but chances are the reasons behind it are unique to you. Before you begin the eating plan, let's take some time to help you get to the root of the issue

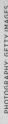

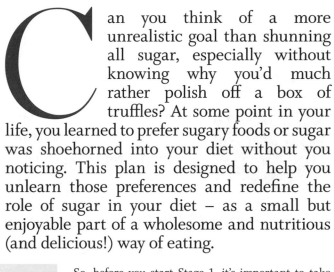

Can you think of a more unrealistic goal than shunning all sugar, especially without knowing why you'd much rather polish off a box of truffles? At some point in your life, you learned to prefer sugary foods or sugar was shoehorned into your diet without you noticing. This plan is designed to help you unlearn those preferences and redefine the role of sugar in your diet – as a small but enjoyable part of a wholesome and nutritious (and delicious!) way of eating.

So, before you start Stage 1, it's important to take a few days to prepare and acclimatise for what lies ahead. Like diving into chilly water, going from a sugar-packed diet to a sugar-smart one in a single leap can be a shock to your system (and make you more likely to leap back out again).

Over the next five days, you'll follow your regular diet as you gradually taper your intake of sugars from all three sources – Straight-Up Sugars, Secret Sugars, and Sugar Mimics. This approach will allow your body and mind time to adjust, and give you the opportunity to really understand the role that sugar plays in your life and your diet.

During the first two days, you'll have exactly the same foods and drink that you normally do, but keep a log of everything you've consumed (and, if possible, in what quantities). On Day 3, you'll use this log to complete an exercise designed to reveal three crucial sides of your unique sugar profile:

- The sugar sources that get to you most
- The emotions that trigger your need for sugar
- Your everyday habits of sugar consumption

During Days 3 to 5, you'll be taking practical action to eliminate sugars from your kitchen and get your fridge, freezer and cupboards ready for Phase 1 of the *Shrink Your Sugar Belly* eating plan.

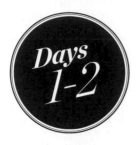

Days 1-2

» **Eat the way you normally do**
» **Explore your relationship with sugar**
» **Keep a food log**

ASSESS The reasons you eat sugar

We can't make this point strongly enough: you're *supposed* to enjoy a chocolate-chip cookie or a bowl of ice cream. We now know how you're hardwired to want sweet foods, so if you swoon for them, you're only following nature's operating manual. And because food is a key part of socialising, we're especially prone when dining out or celebrating special occasions.

But if an out-of-control sweet tooth threatens your health or leads to weight gain that causes emotional pain, it's likely that you're overeating sweet foods for reasons other than pleasure. Two of the most common are stress relief and emotional comfort.

When you're drowning in stress, sugar can seem like the friend who understands. But the relief it offers is temporary and there's a price to pay: you can begin to associate sweet foods with comfort. Gradually, you may turn automatically to that immediate, sweet shot of relief and away from healthier stress-management strategies.

Just as sugary foods can momentarily relieve stress, they can also soothe emotions you may want to suppress or ignore. But when you eat to fill yourself up emotionally, not even the most delectable dessert or starchy comfort food can satisfy emotional hunger.

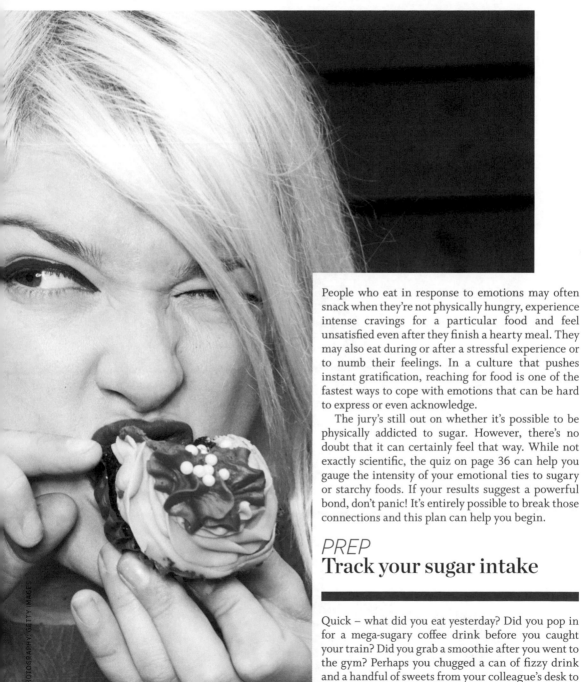

People who eat in response to emotions may often snack when they're not physically hungry, experience intense cravings for a particular food and feel unsatisfied even after they finish a hearty meal. They may also eat during or after a stressful experience or to numb their feelings. In a culture that pushes instant gratification, reaching for food is one of the fastest ways to cope with emotions that can be hard to express or even acknowledge.

The jury's still out on whether it's possible to be physically addicted to sugar. However, there's no doubt that it can certainly feel that way. While not exactly scientific, the quiz on page 36 can help you gauge the intensity of your emotional ties to sugary or starchy foods. If your results suggest a powerful bond, don't panic! It's entirely possible to break those connections and this plan can help you begin.

PREP
Track your sugar intake

Quick – what did you eat yesterday? Did you pop in for a mega-sugary coffee drink before you caught your train? Did you grab a smoothie after you went to the gym? Perhaps you chugged a can of fizzy drink and a handful of sweets from your colleague's desk to get you through the afternoon. Did you nibble on

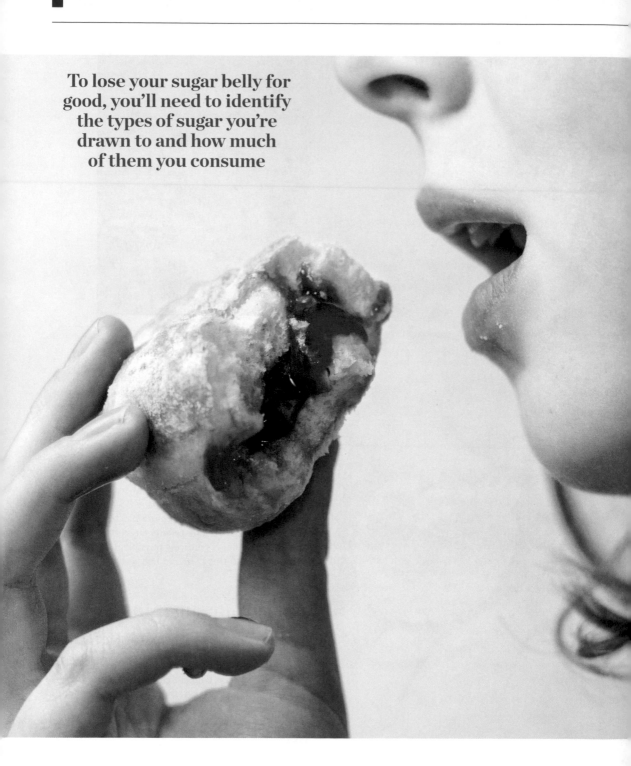

To lose your sugar belly for good, you'll need to identify the types of sugar you're drawn to and how much of them you consume

assessment easy; just jot down the appropriate number. Before you eat, rank your hunger level on a scale of 1 to 5.

Hang on to those logs. You'll be looking at them closely over the next three days. As you do, a picture of your sugar habits will emerge in stark relief. No matter what you discover, the news is good. Once you're aware of your high-sugar preferences – which is not always the case if you eat without thinking – you can swap them for healthier alternatives that are lower in sugar but just as pleasing to your 'sweet buds'.

For example, you might be shocked to find that although you're not a sweets eater, you pack away a ton of foods that act like sugar in your body. Or that your standard café breakfast – scrambled eggs on toast with ketchup – is full of Secret Sugar. Every tablespoon of ketchup contains a teaspoon of added sugar. If you're a woman and use five tablespoons on your breakfast – not hard to do if you don't stay aware of portion sizes – you're consuming practically all of your recommended daily intake of added sugar in ketchup alone.

pretzels while you watched TV? Maybe you made healthy choices all day but blew it with an entire tub of ice cream or a 'Nutella nightcap' (that's the jar and a spoon, by the way) before bed?

We're just guessing here, of course. But to lose your sugar belly for good, you'll need to identify the types of sugar you're drawn to and how much you consume. Record what you eat for breakfast, lunch and dinner and for snacks each day; just for two days.

You may not be a fan of tracking what you eat. Or maybe you just want to stop mucking about and get on with the eating bit. But what you'll discover over this 48-hour period could be revolutionary. Jot down every bite, sip and nibble for just two days. You can simply note what you eat, but if you want more information, add the serving size of each food.

What's key is to track your mood and your hunger level before and after you eat. Both pieces of information are going to tell you a lot about your emotional and physiological connection to sugar. You'll be able to spot patterns that will increase your awareness of what you eat, when you eat and why you choose the foods you do. That's the first step to healthy change. You don't have to write pages and pages. Just a few words will do. See the sample entry on page 34 to get an idea. And we've made the hunger

PHOTOGRAPHY: GETTY IMAGES

HUNGER NUMBERS

Record these values in your eating log to work out what sugar means to you

1   So hungry I'm feeling faint!
2   Audible stomach rumbling
3   Feeling quite hungry, really
4   Yeah, I'd like something to eat
5   I could go without eating for now

Then do the same after you eat:

1   Still hungry. I could eat seconds
2   I'm full, but not quite satisfied
3   I'm pretty content
4   I'm stuffed!
5   I'm so full I feel sick...

DAY ONE

TIME	HUNGRY BEFORE (1-5)	WHAT I ATE	HUNGRY AFTER (1-5)	NOTES

EAT IT, LOG IT

What do you eat normally? And how do you feel about it? Be honest with yourself and these tables could be among the most effective tools in your weight-loss arsenal

MY SUGAR SNAP	WHEN IT STRIKES
Cakes in the office kitchen	*9am, right when I get to work*

DAY TWO

TIME	HUNGRY BEFORE (1-5)	WHAT I ATE	HUNGRY AFTER (1-5)	NOTES

While keeping these records are part of your homework for Days 1-2, feel free to continue charting your progress on the *Shrink Your Sugar Belly* eating plan – and beyond. Every time you eat something, make an entry in the logs above. Add the hunger ratings (see previous page) for before and after you've eaten and when your two days are up you'll be able to examine the motivation behind your sweet treats. But don't just write down what sugary foods you've had, because we'll be examining what sugars are hiding in unexpected places a day or two later... Meanwhile, write down the times that you just know you'll be tempted by sugar – here's where you work out the plan of action that will work best for you, and you alone. Get scribbling!

WHY DO I NEED IT?	MY POSITIVE ALTERNATIVE
Work is so stressful – too much to do and not enough people to help. I'm in a panic most of the day. Plus, I'm always starving when I get to work, and the doughnuts are right there.	*I could make a healthy breakfast at home and eat it at work. I could take a brisk walk around the car park before I enter the building.*

HOW EMOTIONAL IS
YOUR CONNECTION
TO SUGAR?

Think you and sugar might have trouble breaking up? Discover how strong its pull is for you – and what you might expect when you ditch it entirely for Phase 1

1 ***You find it difficult to say no to your favourite sweets.***
Always (add 4 points to column A)
Usually (3 → A)
Sometimes (2 → A)
Rarely or never (2 → B)

2 ***When you've tried to cut back on sugar in the past, how intense were your cravings?***
Very strong You typically ate what you were craving (4 → A)
Strong but more often than not, you were able to satisfy your craving with something healthier than what you wanted (for instance, fruit instead of biscuits) (3 → A)
Noticeable Sometimes you ate what you were craving and sometimes you didn't. (2 →A)
Minor It took some effort, but more often than not, you distracted yourself and the craving passed (1 →B)
Ignorable You were able to get past it pretty easily or you didn't have any cravings (2 →B)

3 ***You often feel guilt or shame after eating sugar.***
Yes (2 →A)
No (2 →B)

4 ***At least one of your favourite sweet treats is fused to a memory of feeling loved and cared for.***
Yes Place a 1 in column A.
No Place a 2 in column B.

5 ***Once you start to eat sugary foods, it's hard to stop.***
Always (5 →A)
Usually (4 →A)
Sometimes (3 →A)
Rarely or never (2 →B)

6 ***Your mood and/or energy level rise right after you eat, but you tend to crash or feel hungry an hour or two later.***
Always or often (3 →A)
Sometimes (2 →A)
Rarely or never (2 →B)

	A	B
1		
2		
3		
4		
5		
6		
7		
8		
9		
10		
11		

Total .... ⊖ ....

Add up your score in each column. Subtract your B score from your A score. ⊜

PHOTOGRAPHY: GETTY IMAGES

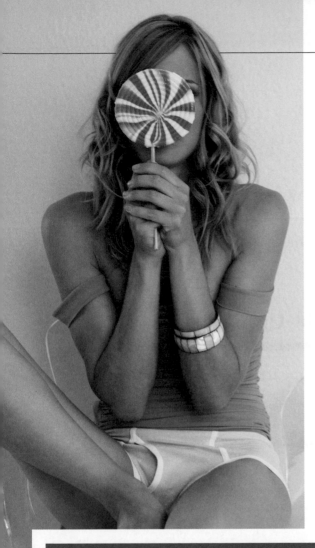

7 *You overeat sugary foods when you're under stress.*
Always or often (3 →A)
Sometimes (2 →A)
Rarely or never (2 →B)

8 *You find yourself thinking about sugary foods ____ times a day.*
More than 4 times (3 →A)
3–4 times (2 →A)
2–3 times (1 →A)
Rarely or never (2 →B)

9 *You seek refuge in sweets to avoid feelings like anger, loneliness, sadness, or powerlessness.*
Always or often (3 →A)
Sometimes (2 →A)
Rarely or never (2 →B)

10 *You reward yourself with sugar after a challenging task – you feel you 'deserve' it.*
Always or often (3 →A)
Sometimes (2 →A)
Rarely or never (2 →B)

11 *The more you indulge in sugar, the less it satisfies – but the more you seem to 'need' it.*
Yes (2 →A)
No (2 →B)

WHAT'S YOUR SUGAR STYLE?

A NEGATIVE NUMBER Your emotional connection to sugar is balanced or non-existent. Wow! But you can still benefit from this book. You might not be aware of how many hidden sugars have crept into your diet.

0–10 You have the odd struggle, but overall keep your cravings pretty much under control. You could still be eating more than you realise, though, and you're likely to notice a difference in the way you feel after following the plan.

11–20 Sugar is one of your go-to coping mechanisms. You may have some withdrawal symptoms as you go through the plan, but will probably spot pleasing results in your weight, cravings and mood by the end of Phase 1.

20+ You're susceptible to sugar's charms, so Phase 1 may be a challenge. Stick with the plan and you will see dramatic results: the *Shrink Your Sugar Belly* eating plan is your answer for emotional equilibrium and a healthy, happy weight.

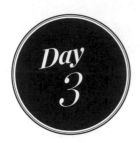

Day 3

» **Eat the way you normally do**
» **Think about your relationship with sugar**
» **Continue with the food log**

ASSESS Your intake of Straight-Up Sugars

Look at your food log. Today you're going to look for entries that contain Straight-Up Sugar – SUS for short. Write this next to each item that you know contains sugar. These foods include:

* Any food or drinks you added sugar to – for instance, a few teaspoons in your coffee or tea or sprinkled onto your cereal in the morning
* Agave syrup, honey, maple syrup
* Sugar-sweetened drinks – fizzy drinks, juices, blended-coffee drinks, lemonades or iced teas, fruit-flavoured drinks, chocolate or strawberry milks, sports drinks
* Jams, chutneys, pickles and preserves
* Chocolate in its many forms – puddings, snack cakes, sweets, cocoa
* Sweets – jelly beans, gummy sweets, licorice, mints
* Sweetened cereals
* Granola or energy bars
* Cookies, doughnuts, snack cakes, muffins, pies and other bakery items
* Cake, muffin or sweet-bread mixes
* Ice cream, sorbet or frozen yoghurt
* Fruit or flavoured yoghurt

Count the number of items and write them down in your log. If you chose to write down your serving sizes, you can estimate the grams of sugar you're getting from these foods. For assistance, look at the item's 'Nutrition' label. Add up the grams and divide by four to get the number of teaspoons of Straight-Up Sugars you typically eat – there are four grams of sugar in one teaspoon. Remember that the eventual goal of the *Shrink Your Sugar Belly* diet is to go on to be eating six to nine teaspoons of added sugar per day. Are you close? Congratulations! If not, don't worry. Use that number as motivation as you go through the plan.

ASSESS
Your sugar preferences

Next, take a close look at all of the Straight-Up Sugars you eat. What time of day did you eat them? How were you feeling when you ate them? (This is where the mood and hunger information on your food log comes in handy.) Are there some you ate out of habit rather than pleasure?

Note any cravings that pop up at the same time each day. For example, let's say you 'need' ice cream after dinner. Noticing – and honouring – such cravings can help you say no to sugary items during the day. You might come to realise that no sugary treats throughout the day come close to satisfying

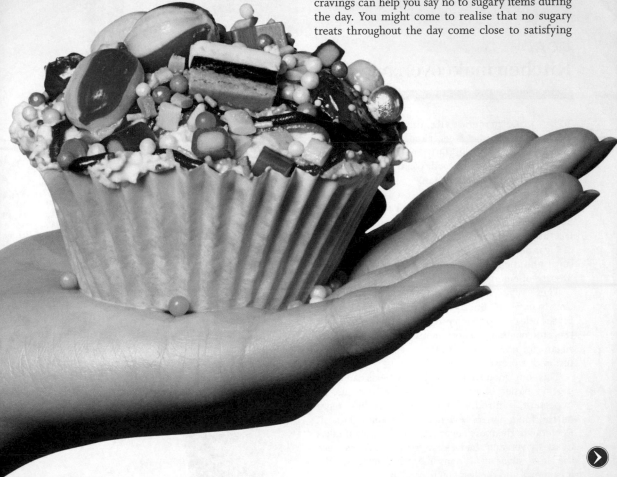

like that nightly dish of ice cream does. (At least for now, while you're still prepping.)

Now for the question we want you to think hardest about: which of the Straight-Up Sugars you marked on your eating log did you really, genuinely enjoy, as opposed to scoffed down without really thinking about it? Or, to put it another way, if you could only have one sweet hit, which one would it be? Maybe a morning without a pastry feels impossible, or you're wedded to your evening ice-cream fix, or you can't do without coffee and a brownie at your desk come 3pm.

You've just identified the one or two favourite treats that are your key sugar sources. Have them, but otherwise don't eat any other Straight-Up Sugars today. And look at the table on the opposite page for alternative options for the three most popular sugar weaknesses for the next three days.

PREP
Kitchen makeover, part 1

Today's task is to remove all of the Straight-Up Sugars lurking in your fridge, freezer and kitchen cupboards. But don't feel too sad! You're making room for the new, deliciously healthy foods you'll soon be enjoying when you start the eating plan.

Start with your fridge first, then move to your freezer and cupboards. Lay out all the Straight-Up Sugar sources on your kitchen tops and take one last look at the cereal bars that pack 25 grams of sugar per serving, the ice-cream syrup that's liquid sugar and the sweets you retrieved from your secret 'in-case-of-emergency' stash.

These sugary seducers have had their shot – it's time to move on. Bin them or give them away, except for the one or two treats you've already chosen, as per the previous page. Those items are your must-have sugars, for now, and you're free to enjoy them for the rest of this preparation period.

This long goodbye to your sugary foods can make it a bit easier to let them go – for now. Just as important, it introduces the idea of 'spending' sugar on the foods where you notice and enjoy it most. Remember, the more sugar you eat, the more it takes to satisfy you and the less of a treat it is. Conversely, the less sugar you consume, the more special it becomes and the less you'll 'need' it.

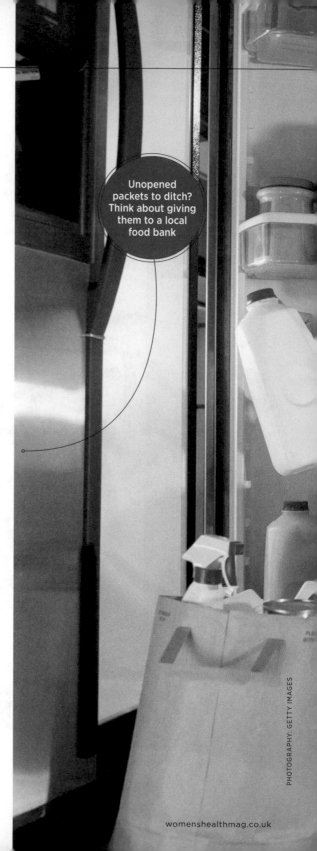

Unopened packets to ditch? Think about giving them to a local food bank

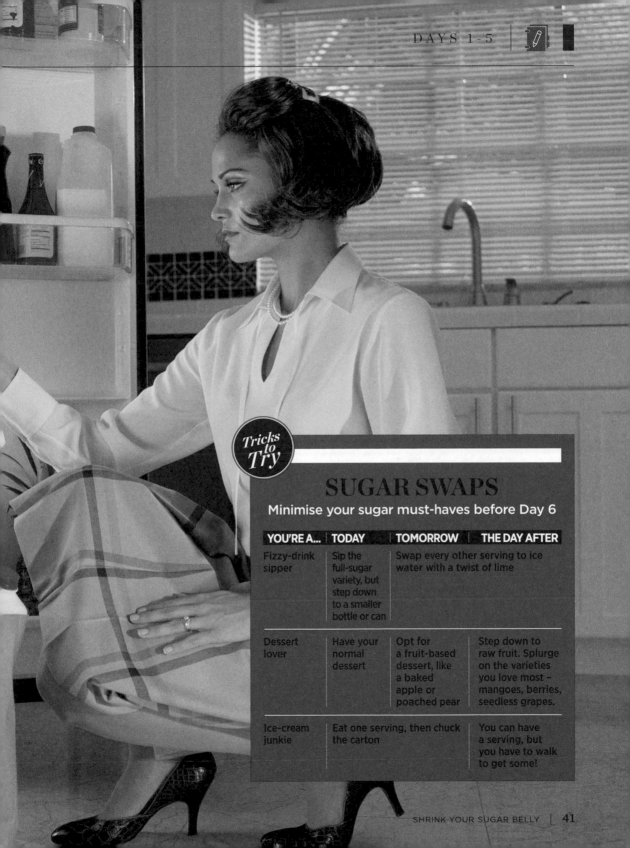

Tricks to Try

SUGAR SWAPS
Minimise your sugar must-haves before Day 6

YOU'RE A...	TODAY	TOMORROW	THE DAY AFTER
Fizzy-drink sipper	Sip the full-sugar variety, but step down to a smaller bottle or can	Swap every other serving to ice water with a twist of lime	
Dessert lover	Have your normal dessert	Opt for a fruit-based dessert, like a baked apple or poached pear	Step down to raw fruit. Splurge on the varieties you love most – mangoes, berries, seedless grapes.
Ice-cream junkie	Eat one serving, then chuck the carton		You can have a serving, but you have to walk to get some!

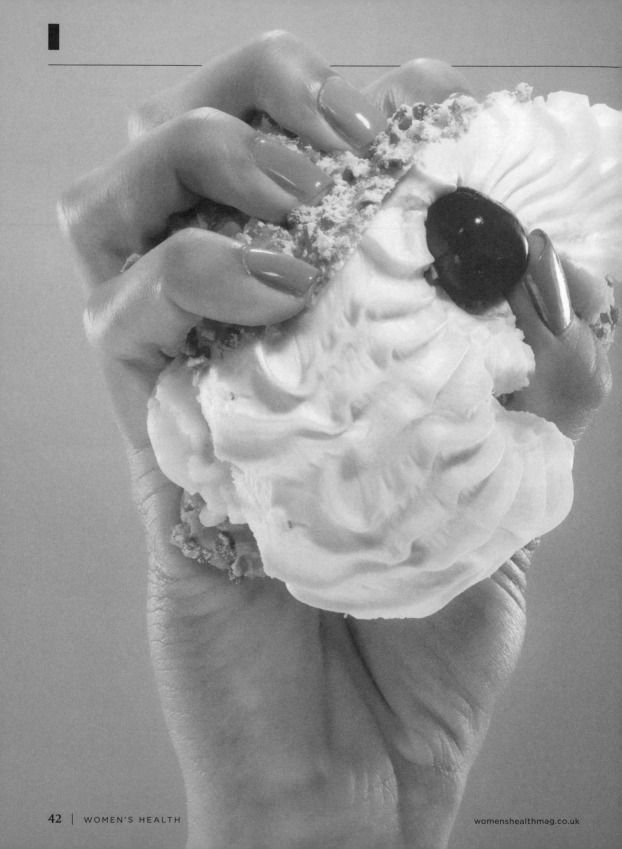

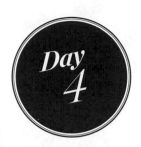

Day 4

» **Uncover your hidden sugar triggers**
» **Spot and eliminate Secret Sugars in your diet**
» **Spot and eliminate Sugar Mimics in your diet**

ASSESS The situations that lead you to reach for sugar

Cravings and food preferences aren't the only things that draw us towards sugar. Habits or external cues are also a factor. Today, you'll look at your typical routine to pinpoint the times and situations that trigger cravings. For instance, how many of us sit down and... just eat – without TV, internet or (naughty!) a bit of work? If you're not one of those rare people, practising mindful eating may help you feel more satisfied, with less sugar.

A study published in the journal *Psychological Science* found that people who eat or drink while they're distracted require far greater intensities of taste – sweetness included – to feel satisfied. In one part of the study, people who made and tasted lemonade as they memorised a seven-digit number ended up with a 50 per cent higher sugar concentration in their drink than when they had to memorise just one number. In other words, a healthy meal may be flavourful and fulfilling if you eat it mindfully, but seem bland if you're distracted with work or TV. And this can prompt you to eat even more sugar after dinner, just to feel satisfied.

Look back at your food log again and think about the triggers that led you to reach for sugar, and jot them down on a chart like the one on pages 34–35. Really try to pinpoint the reason each weak point increases your vulnerability to sugary foods and come up with solutions. Keep these to hand – they're your craving-fighting secret weapons.

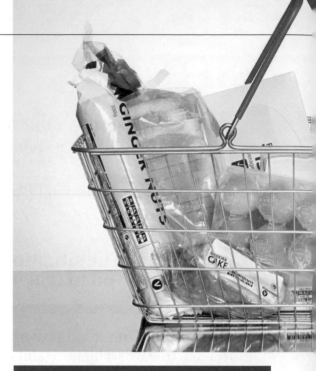

ASSESS
Your intake of Secret Sugars and Sugar Mimics

We've combined Secret Sugars and Sugar Mimics into the same step, because the two categories often come together as a package in foods. Secret Sugars are the ones you wouldn't expect to find in pre-packaged, mostly savoury foods (but also in fruit-based products). Sugar Mimics are substances that aren't sugars, but crash your blood sugar just the same. Just like you did yesterday for Straight-Up Sugars, place an 'SS' – Secret Sugar – next to all the foods that you may not think of as containing added sugar, but that do. Do the same for Sugar Mimics – use 'SM' as your mark. Here's what to look for...

FRIDGE			

The first port of call for the habitual snacker is a prime hideout for undercover sugar agents

FOOD TYPE	SS	SM	
Ketchup, BBQ or other sauces	✓		
Teriyaki sauce, plum sauce or other Asian sauces	✓		
Low-fat or fat-free salad dressings or marinades	✓		
Dips and spreads	✓		
Pasta salad, potato salad or coleslaw	✓	✓	
Pre-packed pastry and pizza dough	✓	✓	
Leftovers from takeaway meals	✓	✓	

FREEZER			

Move into the icy wasteland and lurking in the permafrost are frozen sugars

FOOD TYPE	SS	SM	
Frozen meals (low calorie or otherwise)	✓	✓	
Processed meats (sausages, hot dogs)	✓		
Frozen meat or fish prepared with sauces	✓		
Frozen party snacks/nibbles	✓	✓	
Frozen pizzas	✓	✓	
Frozen bread and rolls	✓	✓	
Pies	✓	✓	

*EVEN THE GRAINS THAT ARE SUGAR FREE AND CONTAIN FIBRE ARE PROCESSED AND CAN SPIKE YOUR BLOOD SUGAR. YOU CAN REINTRODUCE WHOLEGRAIN CEREALS WITH 0 GRAMS SUGAR AND AT LEAST 3 GRAMS FIBRE ON PHASE 2 OF THE PLAN.

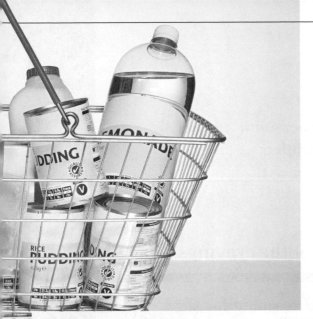

PREP
Kitchen makeover, part 2

Remember what you did yesterday? Do it again! After you review your food log, head to your fridge, freezer and cupboard and find sources of Secret Sugar and Sugar Mimics. But this time, there's an extra step.

Read the ingredients list on the back of the food's package before you make a decision about what to do with it. Look for sugar by one (or more) of its names. Not everything contains them. As for Sugar Mimics, most (eg: wholewheat bread, instant oatmeal and breakfast cereal) contain added sugar as well.

Tortillas, wraps, pitta bread and wholewheat pasta are re-introduced in Phase 2, so you can stash them away until then.

CUPBOARD

Behind the doors, it's a gold mine of Secret Sugars and Sugar Mimics. You'll find them in:

FOOD TYPE	SS	SM		FOOD TYPE	SS	SM	
Crisps, chips or other salty snack foods		✓		Flour, plain or wholewheat		✓	
Pasta sauce	✓			Bread, wholegrain and white	✓	✓	
Pasta, regular and wholewheat		✓		Baked beans	✓		
Couscous, white rice and rice cakes		✓		Trail mix	✓		
Rice mixes	✓	✓		Wholegrain crackers	✓	✓	
Instant flavoured porridge	✓	✓		Toasting muffins	✓	✓	
Cereal or fruit and grain bars (wholegrain varieties included)	✓	✓		Pitta bread, tortilla wraps and taco shells	✓	✓	
Wholegrain cold cereals*	✓	✓		Fruit yoghurt	✓		

Day 5

» **Find your own personal 'rewards'**
» **Eliminate fruit juice**
» **Get ready for Phase 1!**

ASSESS Sugar-free ways to soothe cravings

So, how can you break the cycle of reaching for sugar when emotions strike? The answer lies in finding something to short-circuit that response when you're provoked. When you start on the eating plan in Chapter 3 you'll find a choice of strategies designed to break the connection between your body or brain and sugar. Every day, you can take action to ease stress in the moment and help manage it consistently – and encourage yourself to become aware of negative feelings, so you can learn to manage them without sweets.

As you've learned, there's evidence that highly palatable food – chocolate cake and ice cream definitely qualify – can activate the brain-reward system. And it could be hardwired into your head: research presented at an annual meeting of the US Society for the Study of Ingestive Behavior reported that some people with a personality trait known as 'reward sensitivity' are predisposed to be highly responsive to cues linked with pleasurable food, like TV ads. Turn the tables on your pleasure-seeking brain by creating your own 'rewards card' – a list of non-food treats that give it (and you) the bliss it seeks, without having to reach for the biscuit tin. And that discovery process can be a pleasure in itself.

And you don't have to wait for cravings to take hold before you take some time to make yourself happy. Make sure you pick at least one every day to get yourself into the habit of treating yourself without ending up stuffing yourself.

PHOTOGRAPHY: GETTY IMAGES

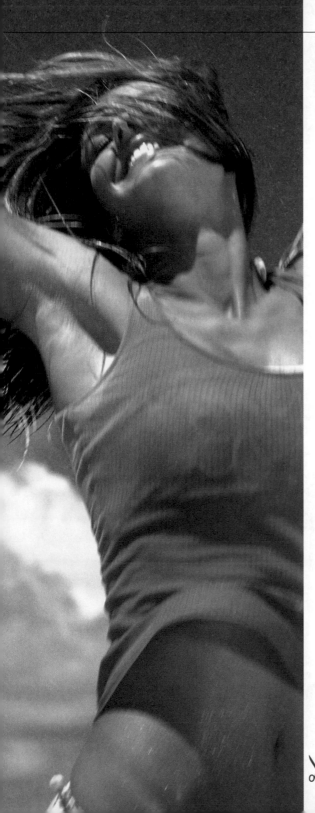

Tricks to Try

YOUR PERSONAL REWARDS CARD

Write down some quick, enjoyable distractions that you love doing – then cut this list out and stick on the fridge for when cravings come knocking. We've started the ball rolling...

1 **Listen to music**
2 **Paint my nails**
3 **Call – yes, call – a mate**
4 **Go for a quick walk**
5 **Spray on some perfume**

1 _____
2 _____
3 _____
4 _____
5 _____
6 _____
7 _____
8 _____
9 _____
10 _____

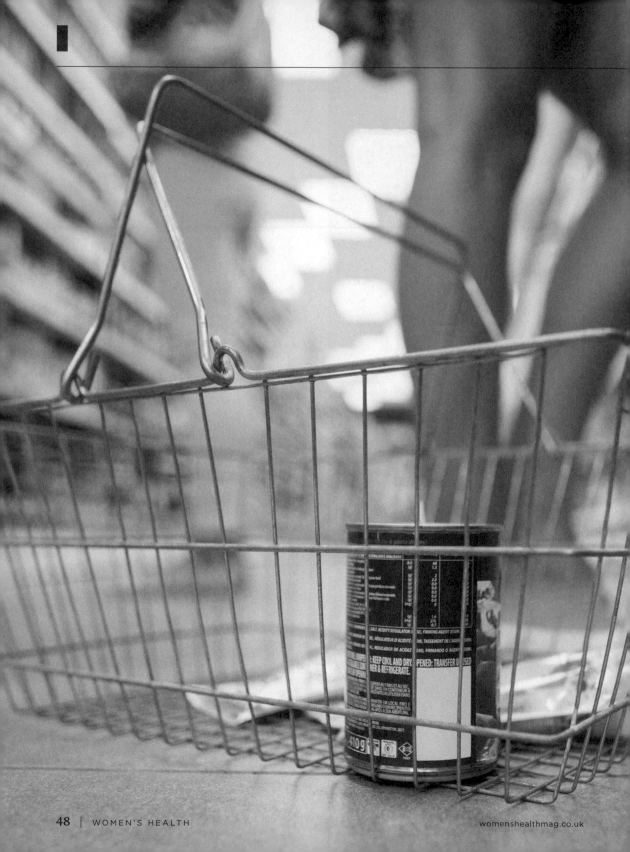

PREP
Shop for reset

Today, you'll be shopping for Phase 1 of the eating plan. Pick out a few of the quick-and-easy meal options from Chapter 3 and start giving those ingredients pride of place in your kitchen.

Put favourite items at eye level. Place vegetables, yoghurt and lean protein in the front and centre of the refrigerator; your pre-popped popcorn and rolled or steel-cut oats on an eye-level kitchen shelf; your package of frozen edamame beans where you can't miss it, so you'll remember to thaw them out in time.

Prep foods for faster meals. As soon as you get home from the supermarket, wash, slice and peel your crudités, avocado and salad vegetables and place them in see-through containers. Boil eggs and prepare grains the night before you plan to eat them. When you get home hungry, you'll be able to whip up a healthy meal without a lot of tedious prep work.

Hide the junk. If you live with someone who won't be eating along with you and the plan, keep their options – especially the sweets and treats – on the bottom shelf of the refrigerator, on the lower shelf in your freezer, and in high or low shelves in your cupboards, where you're less likely to see them.

Don't bulk-buy. Hit the supermarket more often and buy only the next few meals, rather than lay in supplies for the week. An overload of choices at home may deplete your willpower, a *Journal of Consumer Psychology* study found.

You're ready for Phase 1!

Now that you've identified your sugar profile and swapped the sugar bombs in your kitchen with whole, natural foods, you're ready to start your journey to sugar freedom. The first step? Removing all sugar from your diet – temporarily, we promise. We'll stick with you every step of the way, offering practical ways to prevent and relieve cravings and curb any crankiness. The benefits you stand to gain in Phase 1 far outweigh any short-term discomfort you may experience. Less than a week from now, your waistband will be looser, your energy higher, and your mood brighter.

Just as important, you'll have turned your diet around in ways that maybe you didn't think were possible. You'll be passing up your morning pastry and coffee drink, kicking your bottle-a-day cola habit and eliminating those nightly ice-cream fests. That's just for starters. The sweet life is within your grasp; turn the page and reach for it.

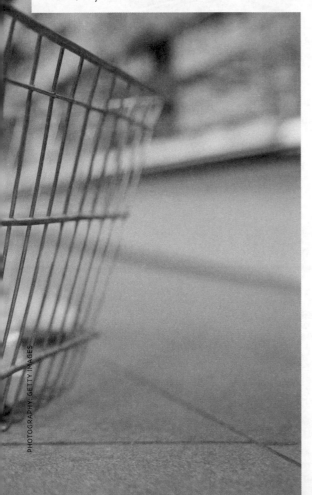

PHOTOGRAPHY: GETTY IMAGES

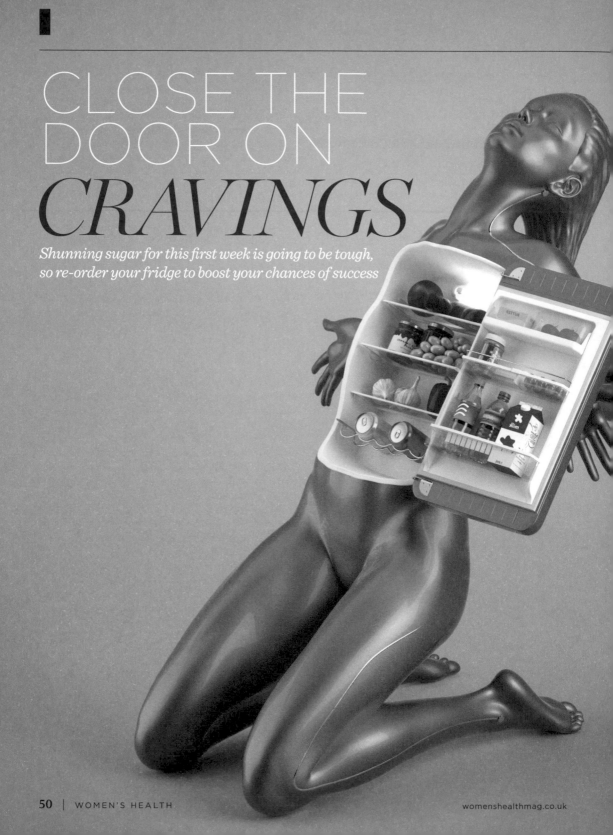

CLOSE THE DOOR ON
CRAVINGS

Shunning sugar for this first week is going to be tough,
so re-order your fridge to boost your chances of success

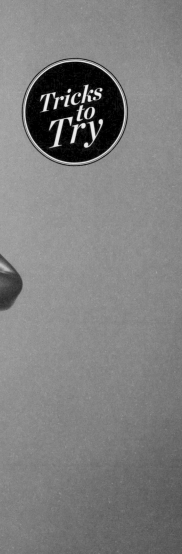

*Tricks
to
Try*

U nless you're one of life's true pedants (or have an overly intimate relationship with your fridge – there is therapy for that sort of thing), chances are you unpack your weekly shop with as much thought as you load Sunday's laundry. A triangle of brie goes slap bang on the top shelf and milk on the inside of the door. Greens and yoghurt might get a slot on the second row, while the slab of chocolate cake – that somehow made it in there – sits glaringly up front. But be warned, new research shows where you put your food can have a big impact on how much you eat, so it's time to become fridge aware. Here's how to stack – and snack – your sugar belly away.

WATCH OUT, RED ALERT

Ever open your fridge and feel like it's an outtake from Channel 4's *The Hoarder Next Door*? We know the feeling. What we bet you didn't know, though, is research published in the *Journal of Consumer Psychology* found a cluttered fridge can quash your willpower. Nutritionist and weight-loss coach Nicky Anstey explains that in a busy fridge, the bright, attractive packaging of less healthy foods distracts you from the more earthy colours of your fresh produce.

There's a reason McDonald's chose a red and yellow colour scheme. Both these colours have been proven to boost your appetite, particularly red, which signals ripeness, sweetness and calories, according to research published in the *Journal of Sensory Studies*. So ditch the strawberry cheesecake and replace it with red- or yellow-hued healthy snacks. Pass the peppers, please.

MAKE EYE CONTACT

"Place your healthiest snacks and food with the most nutrients at eye level," says eating and behavioural therapist James Lamper. "So if you get the munchies, they'll be the first thing you see when you open the fridge." According to a study from Cornell University, you're 2.7 times more likely to eat healthy food if it's in your line of sight. If you want to go the extra mile, store your naughty treats at the very back of the fridge and the bottom of the pile. A study led by nutritional behaviour professor Dr Brian Wansink suggests the more inconvenient the location of your chocolate, the less likely you'll reach for it. How unfortunate.

BUY BIG, EAT SMALL

A study published in the *Journal of Marketing* found people eat larger quantities of junk food if it's kept in clear packages. The same research also showed that when your naughty treats are bite-size, you're more likely to eat them. (Our advice: buy the bowling ball of Edam cheese rather than seductive Mini Babybels). So keep your chocolate and cheese in opaque Tupperware at the back of the fridge. And if you can, make the containers blue. Studies show that blue is an appetite suppressant. Who knew?

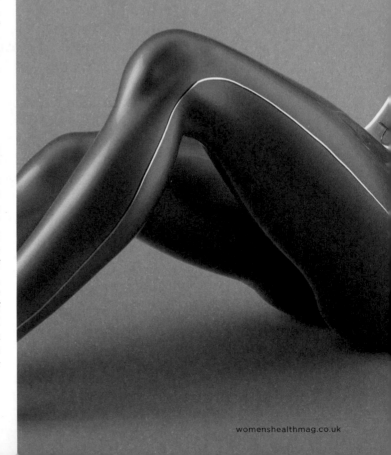

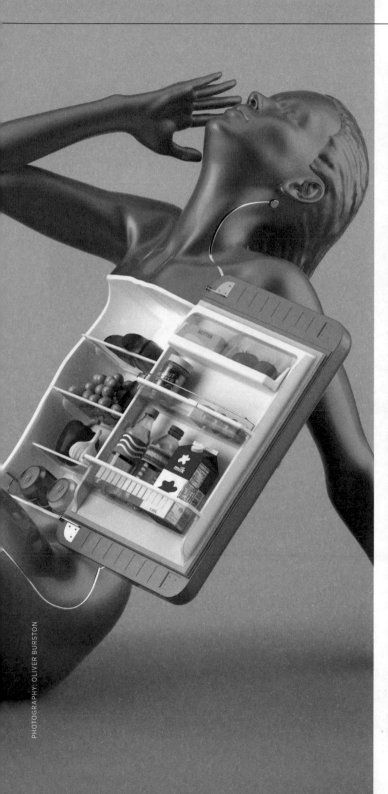

PHOTOGRAPHY: OLIVER BURSTON

CHILL TO PERFECTION

The fridge digits to ramp up your food's nutritional value

2-3°C The ideal temperature of any fridge to keep nasty bacteria at bay. **TIP:** Cold air sinks, so the bottom of the fridge is coolest. Keep your raw meat here.

4-5°C Your non-perishables like butter, jam and eggs need to be in the warmest part of the fridge. **TIP:** Keep them on the top shelf of the fridge door.

13°C Cucumbers taste perfect at this temperature. That's the trick to keeping them crunchy. **TIP:** Wrap them in a tea towel and keep on the top shelf.

21°C Leave watermelon out at room temperature to double its lycopene and betacarotene. **TIP:** Leave it out for a few days; to get that quenching effect leave it in the fridge before eating.

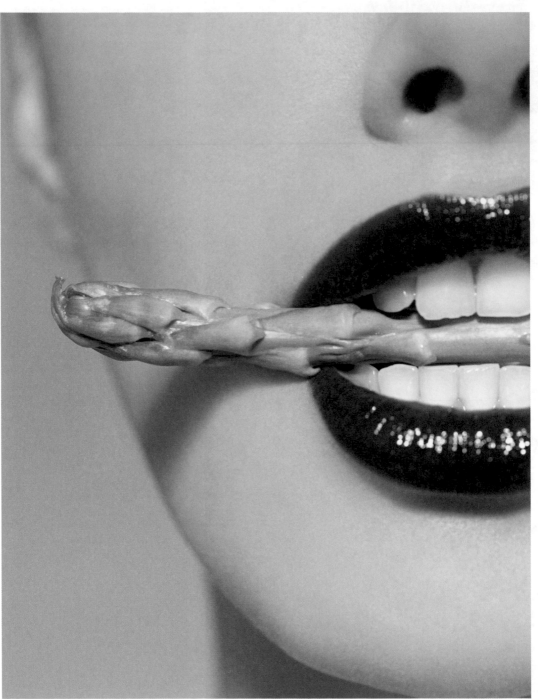

DAYS
6-12

+ BREAKFASTS + LUNCHES + SNACKS +

You've taken stock of your relationship with sugar and started to chip away at it in your everyday diet. What next? That'll be Phase 1, in which you remove the stuff entirely – for now. Tackle withdrawal pangs by filling up on protein-rich breakfasts, then distract your jaded taste buds with high-flavour meals and treats

60 Breakfasts
The secret to keeping cravings at arm's length? It's all about what meal you eat first thing. Lay on the protein and stay fuller for longer.

62 Main meals
Pick what you fancy for your lunch and dinner – or even invent your own dish! – and fend off sweet temptation with a wide range of flavours.

68 Snacks
Avoid blood-sugar dips (and the resulting cravings) between meals when you pack these portable, pick-at-able treats.

74 Stay Energised
Withdrawal from sugar can often leave you listless and cranky – here are seven must-try tricks to reset your pep and keep you on track.

SHRINK YOUR SUGAR BELLY | 55

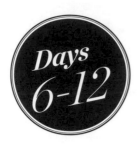

Days 6-12

PHASE ONE:
THE TOUGH-LOVE TURNAROUND

Take a moment to pat yourself on the back. Being that honest with your yourself isn't easy, but hopefully your eyes have been opened. You've gathered crucial intelligence about yourself and the role that sugar plays in your diet – knowledge you're about to put into action to slim your body and safeguard your health.

Now welcome to Phase 1. This is where the going gets tough, but, should you succeed, the pay off will be life changing.

Faced with an unruly sweet tooth that wants what it wants when it wants it – "Doughnut! Now!" – you need to exert the same tough love. During this phase, you will remove sugar from your diet. Even fruit. That's the only way to break sugar's grip on you.

Why no fruit? Fruit is good for you. But you need to re-adjust your palate and get your metabolism running smoothly. That's why we don't want you to have any sugar. To that end, this phase also cuts out a vegetable that rivals fruit in sugar content: sweet

Q: CAN I SWAP INGREDIENTS IN A MEAL?

A: Yes, as long as the ingredients are in the same food group and you are eating phase-appropriate foods. So, for example, you can have brown rice instead of quinoa, mozzarella cheese in place of feta, replace dairy milk with soy milk, chickpeas for kidney beans, green beans for broccoli and chicken for fish, if you like. Be sure to keep your portion sizes about the same, too.

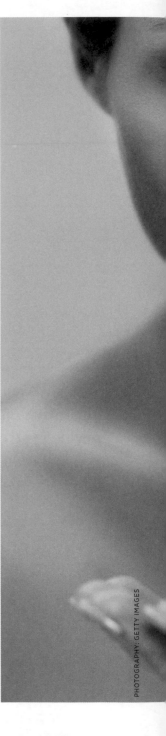

PHOTOGRAPHY: GETTY IMAGES

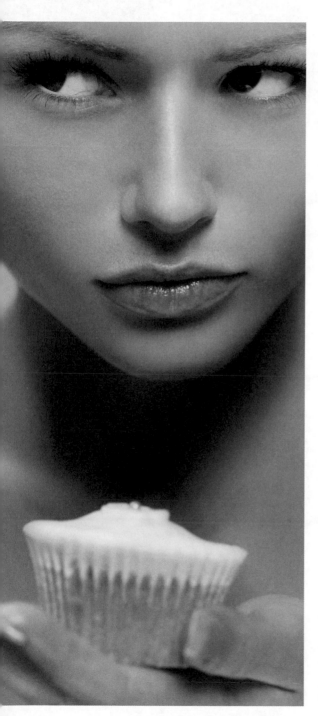

potatoes. Like fruit, it is incredibly nutritious, packed with fibre and antioxidants, and, along with fruit, can come back into your diet when you move on to Phase 2.

To further help you quell cravings, improve the quality of your diet and re-balance the way your body uses glucose and insulin, there are no processed grain products – white or wholewheat – in this phase. Because it can be hard to go without bread or pasta for very long, we begin to bring them back in Phase 2 in limited amounts. However, you don't have to eat them if you don't want to.

We can't sugar-coat it: we call this phase the Tough-love Turnaround because we know that it may not be easy. But we promise you'll love the results! For the first several days, you may not feel at your best, physically or emotionally. Did you ever give up smoking? Do you remember the tiredness and irritability? You may experience similar symptoms, such as headaches, fatigue and edginess, and the cravings may get intense.

Your score on the quiz you completed on Day 1 or 2 (page 36) will give you an indication of how strong your sugar cravings are likely to be. But don't let that scare you – let it be a motivation. The good news: it's all over in seven days and the meals you'll be eating are designed to keep you satisfied, keep your blood-sugar levels steady and keep cravings at bay. All of the meals and recipes were developed with the right balance of protein, carbohydrates and fat to prevent

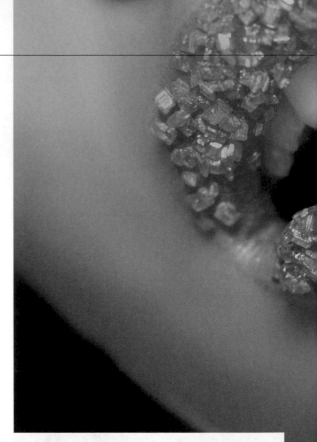

the wild swings in blood sugar and insulin that trigger cravings and promote fat storage.

We've included a daily food log with all of your options on Phase 1 – check off what you eat each day. Plus, this is where our smart tips and your own personal reward card will become an essential part of keeping your motivation on track. And because you'll carry the strategies you learn each day into the next, your discomfort eases day by day. Any symptoms you may experience typically fade, replaced by a positive upswing in energy and mood.

By Day 9, you should begin to notice just how good you feel. More energy, a brighter mood and sound sleep are just the start. As your body regains its sensitivity to insulin and maintains steadier blood-sugar levels, sugar's iron grip on your body and mind will loosen.

So will your waistband. By Day 12, if you've followed the meal plan faithfully, you can expect to lose an average of seven pounds and nearly eight inches all over, nearly two inches from your waist and hips, and an inch off your thighs. Those numbers aren't theoretical – they're the average losses experienced by our test panellists. Women just like you, who shrank their sugar bellies and retrained

SNAP A PHOTO, SNAP OUT OF TEMPTATION

Did you know that taking a photo of every meal or snack before you eat it helps stop over-eating?

In a study published in the *International Journal of Consumer Studies*, participants were asked to keep a written food diary and snap their meals and snacks for a week.

The results? Some liked the photos, some preferred the diary. But everyone said that the photos, and the act of taking them, made them think about what they were eating in a way that the paper diaries didn't. They often adjusted their choices once they'd seen the photo – and thought twice before tucking in.

That minute of delay might just be all you need to decide that you've served up too much, or that you could choose a better option.

While you're at it, try sharing daily photos of your meals and snacks with supportive friends on Instagram – there's no effort like a team effort.

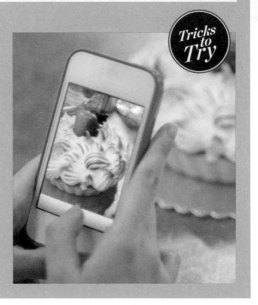

Tricks to Try

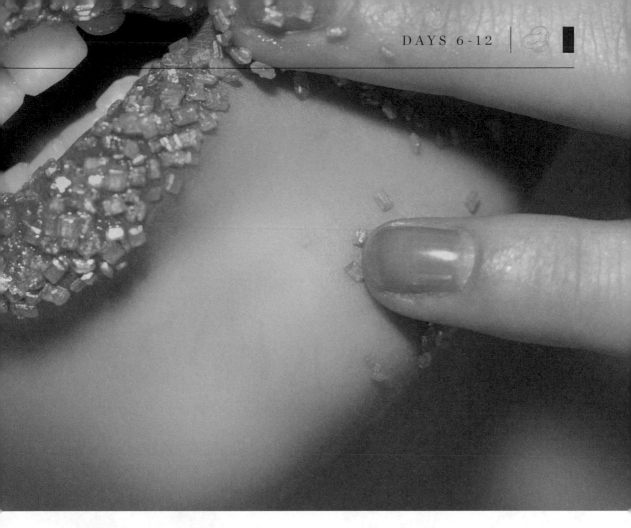

their taste buds to savour the sweetness of whole, natural foods. These rewards aren't temporary, like a sugar buzz. They're lasting and the benefits only get better as you progress through the plan.

DAYS 6-12: **What to do**

Have breakfast every morning to keep cravings at bay. Choose from the high-protein options you'll find on pages 60-61. Breakfasts have about 300 calories and at least 15 grams of protein.

Mix-and-match the lunch and dinner options; they're interchangeable from a calorie and a nutritional perspective. Lunches and dinners contain 400 to 450 calories and, of course, they contain no added sugar. Have something different every day, or stick to three or four meals you love – it's up to you. Every meal is easy and quick to prepare.

Don't forget to snack! Eating every few hours prevents the blood-sugar dips that trigger appetite and sugar cravings. When you have the snacks is up to you. You can snack mid-morning to tide you over until lunch or in the afternoon to keep you going until dinner. Just make sure you're eating something about every four hours.

Avoid the following items: fruit, fruit juice, dried fruit, sweet potatoes, processed grain products (both white and wholewheat) and sugar in any of its many forms (including the table sugar you might add to foods, honey and maple syrup).

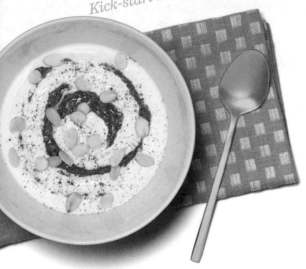

MICROWAVE PEANUT-BUTTER OATS

In a medium microwaveable bowl, mix 240ml skimmed **milk** (or unsweetened **soy milk**), 50g **rolled oats** and a pinch of **salt**. Microwave on high for 2 minutes, then stir in 2 tsps natural **almond** or **peanut butter** and **ground cinnamon** to taste. Microwave on high for another 30 seconds, or until oats are soft. Stir before eating.

Serves 1 | **Ready in** 5 mins
300 **cals** | 2g **sat fat**

Phase One
BREAKFASTS
Kick-start a crave-free day by filling up on these protein-heavy dishes

CRUNCHY ALMOND YOGHURT

Stir 1 tbsp **natural almond** or **peanut butter** into 240g **fat-free plain yoghurt** until smooth. Gently stir in 2 tbsps sliced **almonds** and **ground cinnamon** to taste.

Serves 1 | **Ready in** 3 mins | 311 **cals** | 2g **sat fat**

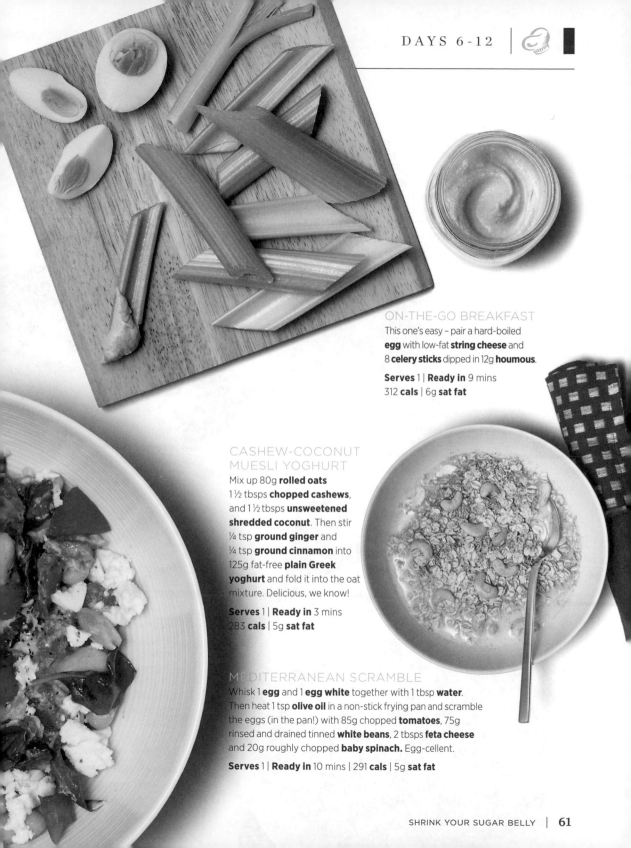

ON-THE-GO BREAKFAST

This one's easy – pair a hard-boiled **egg** with low-fat **string cheese** and 8 **celery sticks** dipped in 12g **houmous**.

Serves 1 | **Ready in** 9 mins
312 **cals** | 6g **sat fat**

CASHEW-COCONUT MUESLI YOGHURT

Mix up 80g **rolled oats** 1½ tbsps **chopped cashews**, and 1½ tbsps **unsweetened shredded coconut**. Then stir ¼ tsp **ground ginger** and ¼ tsp **ground cinnamon** into 125g fat-free **plain Greek yoghurt** and fold it into the oat mixture. Delicious, we know!

Serves 1 | **Ready in** 3 mins
283 **cals** | 5g **sat fat**

MEDITERRANEAN SCRAMBLE

Whisk 1 **egg** and 1 **egg white** together with 1 tbsp **water**. Then heat 1 tsp **olive oil** in a non-stick frying pan and scramble the eggs (in the pan!) with 85g chopped **tomatoes**, 75g rinsed and drained tinned **white beans**, 2 tbsps **feta cheese** and 20g roughly chopped **baby spinach.** Egg-cellent.

Serves 1 | **Ready in** 10 mins | 291 **cals** | 5g **sat fat**

VEGETARIAN STUFFED PORTOBELLO

Makes 4 servings. Prep time: 15 mins. Total time: 40 mins

✳ 4 **portobello mushrooms** ✳ 2 tbsps **olive oil**, divided ✳ 45g **pine nuts**, toasted ✳ ½ block **extra-firm tofu**, drained and cubed ✳ 60g **onion**, chopped ✳ 2 cloves **garlic**, crushed ✳ 2 **tomatoes**, chopped ✳ 60g **fresh spinach**, chopped ✳ 1 tsp **dried basil** ✳ 400g **cooked brown rice** ✳ 1 **egg white**, lightly beaten ✳ ¼ tsp **freshly ground black pepper** ✳ 2 tbsps shredded **Parmesan cheese** ✳ 85g **low-fat mozzarella cheese**, shredded ✳ 3 tbsps chopped **fresh basil**

1/ Pre-heat the oven to 190°C and coat a baking tray with cooking spray.
2/ Cut the stems off the mushrooms and brush the top of each one with a little oil.
3/ Heat the remaining oil in the same frying pan. Add the tofu, onion and garlic. Cook, stirring frequently, for 5 minutes. Then chuck in the tomatoes, spinach and dried basil, and cook for 3 minutes before removing it from the heat.
4/ Stir in the rice, egg white, pepper, Parmesan and ⅓ of the mozzarella. Spoon ¼ of the rice mixture onto each mushroom. Top with the remaining mozzarella and the fresh basil. Place the mushrooms, stuffing side up, on the baking tray and bake for 15 minutes – or until they smell fantastic and the cheese is bubbly.

Serves 2 | **Ready in** 25 mins | 395 **cals** | 5g **sat fat**

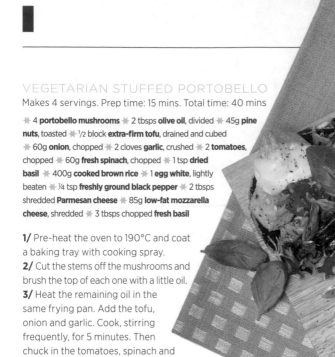

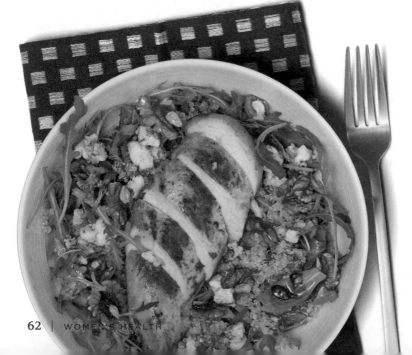

BLUE CHEESE, WALNUT, CHICKEN, AND QUINOA SALAD

Grab a pan and gently cook 40g **rocket leaves** (no, that's not a typo!) and ¼ tsp of **salt** in ½ tsp **olive oil** for 3 minutes, or until wilted. Then whisk up 1 tsp olive oil, ½ tsp **crushed garlic,** and 1 tbsp **balsamic vinegar**. Toss the rocket with 60g cooked **quinoa** and top with 85g **roasted skinless chicken breast** and 2 tsps chopped **walnuts**. The final touches? Drizzle on the **dressing** and 2 tsps crumbled **blue cheese**. Now, doesn't that look good?

Serves 1 | **Ready in** 20 mins
450 **cals** | 3g **sat fat**

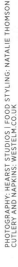

PHOTOGRAPHY: HEARST STUDIOS | FOOD STYLING: NATALIE THOMSON CUTLERY AND NAPKINS: WESTELM.CO.UK

FIESTA EGG SALAD

Mash ¼ **avocado** with 2 tsps **lemon juice**, a pinch each of **ground cumin** and **black pepper**. Mix with 1 hard-boiled **egg** and 1 boiled **egg white**, both chopped. Toss with 240g rinsed and drained tinned **black beans** and 3 tbsps tomato **salsa**. Serve over 60g **baby spinach leaves**. Heaven on a plate...

Serves 1 | **Ready in** 10 mins
416 **cals** | 3g **sat fat**

Phase One
MAIN MEALS

These flavour-filled dishes are double duty. Lunch or dinner? You choose

TANGY MEDITERRANEAN TUNA SALAD

This one's a quickie: whisk together 1½ tsps **olive oil**, 1½ tsps **red-wine vinegar**, ¼ tsp **crushed garlic** and ½ tsp **Dijon mustard**. Gently mix 70g tinned water-packed **tuna** (drained) with 200g tinned **chickpeas** (rinsed and drained), and toss with the dressing. Stir in 2 tbsps sliced **black olives** and serve over 100g of torn **romaine lettuce**.

Serves 1 | **Ready in** 5 mins
453 **cals** | 2g **sat fat**

CRUNCHY SESAME CHICKEN AND BULGUR BOWL

You're ten minutes away from lunchtime bliss: whisk 2 tsps toasted **sesame oil**, 1 tbsp **rice-wine vinegar**, ½ tsp **minced garlic** and ¼ tsp **low-salt soy sauce**. Using a fork, shred an 85g grilled, skinless **chicken breast**. Toss 200g cooked **bulgur** with 60g roughly chopped **spinach**. Top with 2 tbsps chopped **spring onion**, 220g **shredded carrot**, the shredded chicken and 1 tbsp chopped, roasted, salted **peanuts**. Drizzle with the **dressing**. Looks just like the photo (right), doesn't it?

Serves 1 | **Ready in** 10 mins | 447 **cals** | 3g **sat fat**

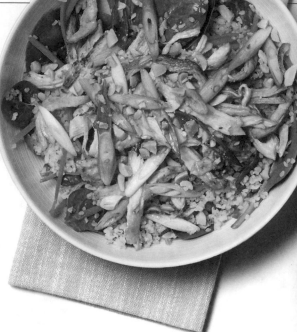

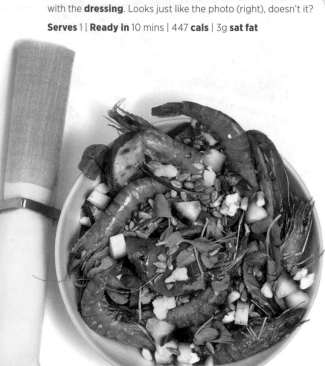

MUSTARD SALMON WITH BROCCOLI AND QUINOA

Mix ¼ tsp each of **crushed garlic**, **dried oregano** and **balsamic vinegar**, plus 1 tsp **Dijon mustard** to make a glaze. Spread it onto an 85g **salmon fillet**. Then sprinkle a pinch of **salt** and **pepper** and 2 tsps **olive oil** over 150g **broccoli florets** laid out on a baking tray. Bake the broccoli at 190°C for 20 minutes, then turn it over before adding the salmon to the tray. While cooking, flip the broccoli and salmon every 3 minutes, until the salmon is just cooked throughout. Serve the fish over 150g cooked quinoa with broccoli on the side. Dig in!

Serves 1 | **Ready in** 30 mins | 436 **cals** | 2g **sat fat**

GRILLED PRAWN SALAD WITH POTATO, SUNFLOWER SEEDS AND GOAT'S CHEESE

Ready, steady, cook! Cut a **potato** into wedges, toss with 1 tsp **olive oil**, a pinch of **salt** and **black pepper**, and bake at 190°C for 25 minutes or until soft on the inside. Then toss 110g **large prawns** with ½ tsp olive oil and 1 tsp **garlic powder**. Grill for 2 minutes on each side until they're pink. Then in a small bowl, whisk 1 tsp olive oil, 1 tbsp **balsamic vinegar** and ¼ tsp **crushed garlic**. Toss 80g **mixed greens** with 60g chopped **cucumber** and the dressing you just made. Top with the prawns, potato, 2 tsps roasted and salted sunflower seeds, and 2 tsps crumbled goat's cheese. Your pals will get food envy!

Serves 1 | **Ready in** 35 mins 477 **cals** | 4g **sat fat**

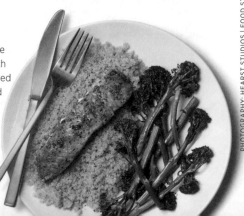

PHOTOGRAPHY: HEARST STUDIOS | FOOD STYLING: NATALIE THOMSON CUTLERY AND NAPKINS: WESTELM.CO.UK

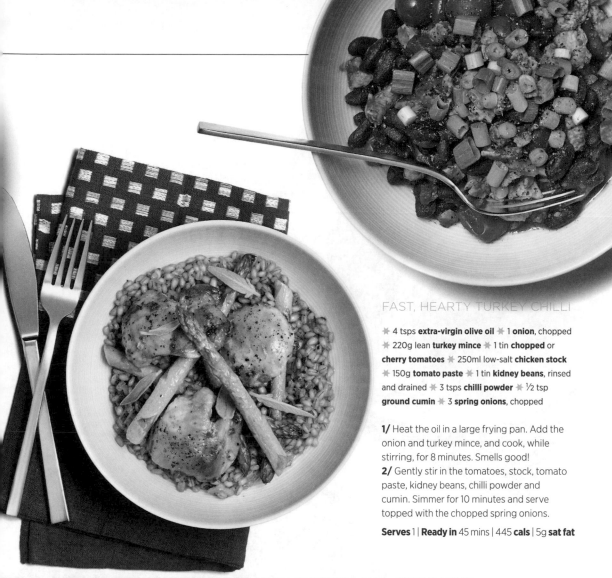

FAST, HEARTY TURKEY CHILLI

✷ 4 tsps **extra-virgin olive oil** ✷ 1 **onion**, chopped
✷ 220g lean **turkey mince** ✷ 1 tin **chopped** or
cherry tomatoes ✷ 250ml low-salt **chicken stock**
✷ 150g **tomato paste** ✷ 1 tin **kidney beans**, rinsed
and drained ✷ 3 tsps **chilli powder** ✷ ½ tsp
ground cumin ✷ 3 **spring onions**, chopped

1/ Heat the oil in a large frying pan. Add the
onion and turkey mince, and cook, while
stirring, for 8 minutes. Smells good!
2/ Gently stir in the tomatoes, stock, tomato
paste, kidney beans, chilli powder and
cumin. Simmer for 10 minutes and serve
topped with the chopped spring onions.

Serves 1 | **Ready in** 45 mins | 445 **cals** | 5g **sat fat**

BARLEY RISOTTO WITH CHICKEN AND ASPARAGUS

✷ 3 tbsps **lemon juice** ✷ ¼ tsp **salt** ✷ 1 clove **garlic**, crushed ✷ 4 tsps **olive oil** ✷ 450g **boneless, skinless chicken thighs** ✷ 450g **asparagus**, ends trimmed ✷ 1.1L **vegetable broth** ✷ 1 **onion**, chopped ✷ 1 **shallot**, chopped ✷ 2 tbsps **dried sage leaves** ✷ ¼ tsp **black pepper** ✷ 40g **pearl barley**

1/ Find your large saucepan and chopping board, pre-heat
the oven to 200°C and line a baking tray with foil.
2/ In a large bowl, whisk the lemon juice, salt, garlic,
and 1 tsp of the oil. Mix in the chicken and asparagus.
3/ Place the chicken on the baking tray and cook
for 25 minutes. Add the asparagus to the baking tray
during the final 10 minutes of the chicken's cooking time.
4/ While your meat is in the oven, pour the broth into
a saucepan, cook for 5 minutes, then remove from the heat.
5/ Heat the remaining oil in a large saucepan. Add the onion

and shallot and cook for 5 minutes, stirring. Throw in the
sage and black pepper, and cook for 1 minute, then lower the
heat, stir in the barley and cook for another 2 minutes.
6/ Add a little broth to the barley – around 200ml; simmer
and allow the barley to soak up the liquid, then add a little
more broth. Continue this process until all of the broth
is absorbed and the barley is tender and creamy.
7/ Remove the saucepan from the heat. Serve the barley
risotto topped with the chicken and asparagus. Delicious!
Serves 2 | **Ready in** 45 mins | 467 **cals** | 4g **sat fat**

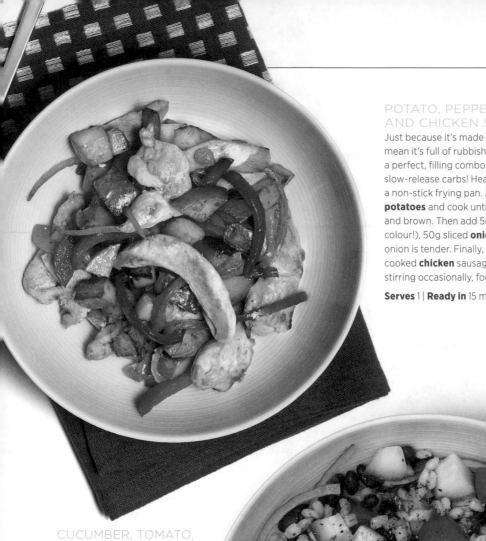

POTATO, PEPPER AND CHICKEN SAUTÉ

Just because it's made in a frying pan, doesn't mean it's full of rubbish. This recipe packs a perfect, filling combo of protein and slow-release carbs! Heat 2 tsps **olive oil** in a non-stick frying pan. Add 150g chopped **potatoes** and cook until they begin to soften and brown. Then add 50g sliced **pepper** (any colour!), 50g sliced **onion** and cook until the onion is tender. Finally, add 1 finely chopped, cooked **chicken** sausage (yum!) and cook, stirring occasionally, for another 4 minutes.

Serves 1 | **Ready in** 15 mins | 412 **cals** | 3g **sat fat**

PHOTOGRAPHY: HEARST STUDIOS. | FOOD STYLING: NATALIE THOMSON
CUTLERY AND NAPKINS: WESTELM.CO.UK

CUCUMBER, TOMATO, BLACK BEAN AND BARLEY SALAD

Grab a fork and whisk 1 tbsp **red-wine vinegar**, 2 tsps **olive oil**, ¼ tsp **dried oregano** and ½ tsp **crushed garlic**. (Go on, give it some elbow grease.) Then toss 90g halved **plum tomatoes**, 60g chopped **cucumber**, 2 tbsps finely chopped **red onion**, 80g cooked **barley**, 80g tinned **black beans** (rinsed and drained). Pop the dressing on, then it's good to tuck in!

Serves 1 | **Ready in** 20 mins
449 **cals** | 3g **sat fat**

BUILD YOUR OWN...

Live life (or at least lunchtime) on the edge by taking the recipe into your own hands. To make a tasty, healthy, sugar-smart meal, simply mix-and match an ingredient from each of the categories below.

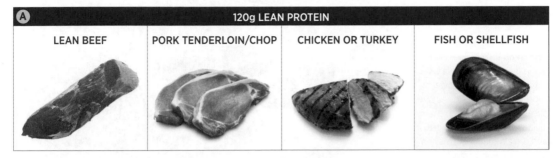

A **120g LEAN PROTEIN**

| LEAN BEEF | PORK TENDERLOIN/CHOP | CHICKEN OR TURKEY | FISH OR SHELLFISH |

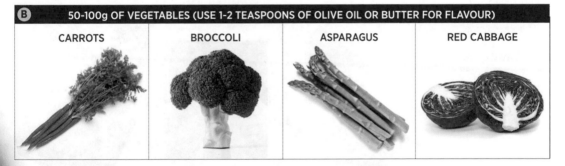

B **50-100g OF VEGETABLES (USE 1-2 TEASPOONS OF OLIVE OIL OR BUTTER FOR FLAVOUR)**

| CARROTS | BROCCOLI | ASPARAGUS | RED CABBAGE |

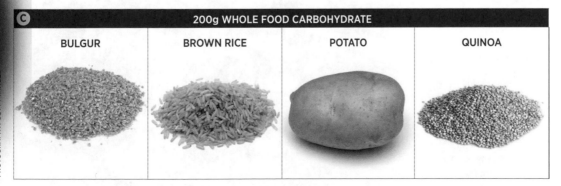

C **200g WHOLE FOOD CARBOHYDRATE**

| BULGUR | BROWN RICE | POTATO | QUINOA |

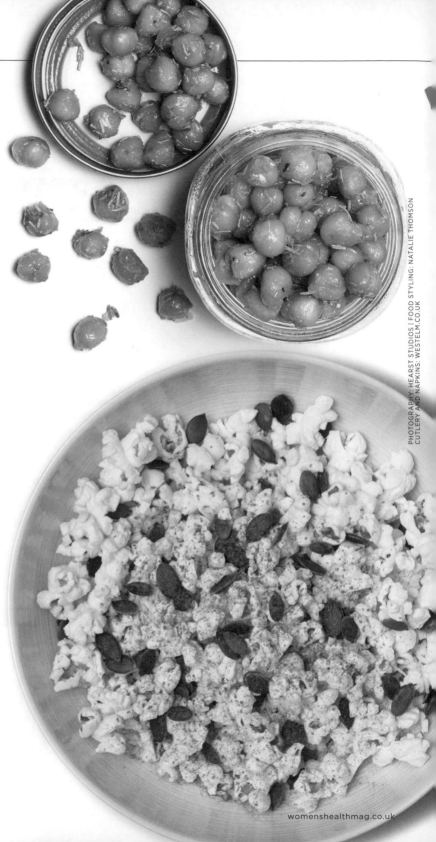

PHOTOGRAPHY: HEARST STUDIOS | FOOD STYLING: NATALIE THOMSON
CUTLERY AND NAPKINS: WESTELM.CO.UK

CRUNCHY ROASTED ROSEMARY CHICKPEAS

* 1 tin **chickpeas**, rinsed and drained
* 1½ tbsps **olive oil**
* ¼ tsp **garlic powder**
* 1½ tsps **dried rosemary**
* ¼ tsp **salt**

1/ Pre-heat the oven to 200°C.
2/ Spread the chickpeas on a paper towel in a single layer. Place another paper towel on top and gently dab to remove excess water. Then pop the chickpeas onto a baking tray and drizzle the oil on, tossing them with your hands to ensure they are all coated well.
3/ Spread the chickpeas into a single layer again and bake for 15 minutes. Give them a stir and shake, then place them in the oven for another 10 minutes, until they're golden and crisp.
4/ Remove the chickpeas from the oven and toss with the garlic powder, rosemary and salt. Easy peas-y!

Serves 1 | **Ready in** 30 mins
130 **cals** | 1g **sat fat**

POPCORN AND PUMPKIN SEED MIX

In a pot (with a lid!), air-pop 10g **popcorn kernels** according to the packet instructions. Leave to cook, then sprinkle with 2 tbsps **pumpkin seeds**, 1 tsp **unsweetened coconut** and a pinch of **ground cinnamon**. Now, which DVD to watch...?

Serves 1 | **Ready in** 20 mins
153 **cals** | 5g **sat fat**

CASHEW-GINGER COCONUT MUESLI

This one's straightforward, but we'll share the recipe anyway: put 2 tbsps **rolled oats**, 1 tbsp **cashews**, 1 tbsp **unsweetened shredded coconut**, ⅛ tsp each of **ground ginger** and **ground cinnamon** into a bowl. Then add 70ml **skimmed milk** and stir well. Zap it in the microwave for 2 minutes, if you prefer hot, softer oats. Snack happy.

Serves 1 | **Ready in** 2 mins
155 **cals** | 5g **sat fat**

SNACKS
Phase One

Dodge between-meal cravings – pick two a day

CHEESY POPCORN WITH ALMONDS

You know what to do: in a pot, air-pop 10g **popcorn kernels**. Then sprinkle with **Parmesan cheese** and 16 **almonds**.

Serves 1 | **Ready in** 10 mins
161 **cals** | 2g **sat fat**

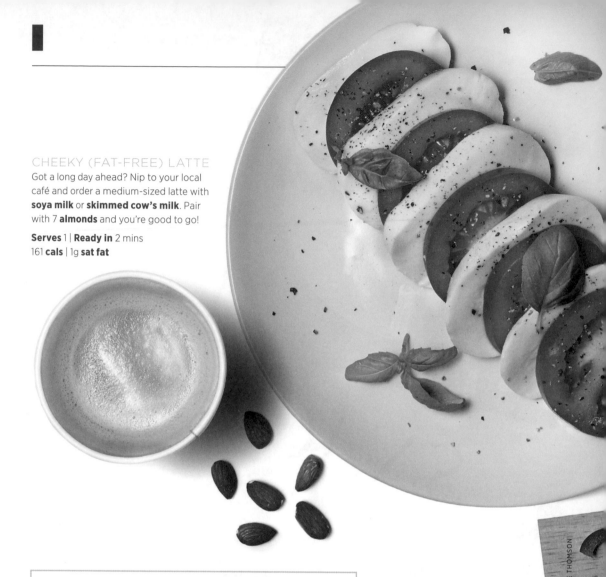

CHEEKY (FAT-FREE) LATTE

Got a long day ahead? Nip to your local café and order a medium-sized latte with **soya milk** or **skimmed cow's milk**. Pair with 7 **almonds** and you're good to go!

Serves 1 | **Ready in** 2 mins
161 **cals** | 1g **sat fat**

TAKE A STANCE AGAINST SUGAR

Chase off cravings with yoga – it'll help quiet the chatterings in your mind and help you make friends with your body again. There are two routines for you to try on pages 118-127, or for a full body-and-mind workout, seek out a hatha yoga session. The most common type of yoga practiced in the UK, hatha is made up of poses, breathing techniques to help tame your stress response, and meditation to help you to tune in to desires that sweet treats can't satisfy.

TURKEY, CHEESE AND VEGETABLES

Simply have a little munch on 60g thinly sliced **deli turkey**, 175g **red pepper**, sliced, and 1 **string cheese** to graze away future cravings.

Serves 1 | **Ready in** 1 min
159 **cals** | 4g **sat fat**

PHOTOGRAPHY: HEARST STUDIOS. FOOD STYLING: NATALIE THOMSON. CUTLERY AND NAPKINS: WESTELM.CO.UK

CAPRESE

This classic never fails to hit the spot. Slice a beef **tomato** and top with the following: **fresh basil** (or a fresh or dried herb of your choice), a pinch of **salt**, **ground pepper** to taste and 1 tsp **olive oil**. Serve with 30g fresh, sliced **mozzarella**.

Serves 1 | **Ready in** 2 mins
195 **cals** | 3g **sat fat**

GO GREEN

No matter what phase of the Sugar Smart Diet plan you're on, drinking green tea is a tasty, natural way to manage your blood sugar, according to an analysis of 17 studies of green tea published in the *American Journal of Clinical Nutrition*. It linked this fragrant tea to lowering both fasting levels of blood sugar and levels of HbA1c, which indicates the presence of long-term glucose in the blood. One study even found that green tea increases the body's ability to burn fat! Studies have show that four cups a day brings the most benefit. Stick that kettle on!

PB, CELERY AND MILK

Another grazey one – *but* you burn more calories eating the celery than it contains because it's so crunchy. Spread a tbsp of natural **peanut butter** onto 4 **celery** sticks, then dip in 100ml **skimmed milk**.

Serves 1 | **Ready in** 2 mins
146 **cals** | 2g **sat fat**

YOUR PHASE 1 EATING LOG

	BREAKFAST	SNACK	LUNCH	SNACK
Day 7				
Day 8				
Day 9				
Day 10				
Day 11				
Day 11				
Day 12				

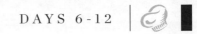

DINNER	WORKOUT	TIPS I TRIED	HOW I FEEL

7 WAYS TO STAY ENERGISED DURING PHASE ONE

How's your energy? If you're flagging a bit, don't panic. You may be experiencing sugar 'withdrawal', which can cause some people to experience temporary fatigue or mental fogginess. While some people will breeze through Phase One, others might well feel a bit pooped, especially in those first few sugar-free days. If this sounds like you, these mind-and-body tips can help perk up both your body and your brain. And hang in there; the fatigue will pass. In fact, you should feel more energised as time goes on.

1

Revive with rosemary

It isn't just for lamb: the fresh herb's pleasant, spicy scent is a literal eye-opener, suggests a study published in the *International Journal of Neuroscience*. Researchers gave 40 volunteers EEGs, which measure the brain's electrical activity, then had them smell rosemary for 3 minutes both before and after they completed a simple maths test.

The volunteers' EEGs showed the reduction of certain brain waves in the frontal cortex, which indicates increased alertness. Keep a small bottle of rosemary essential oil in your bag and when that mental fog rolls in... just inhale.

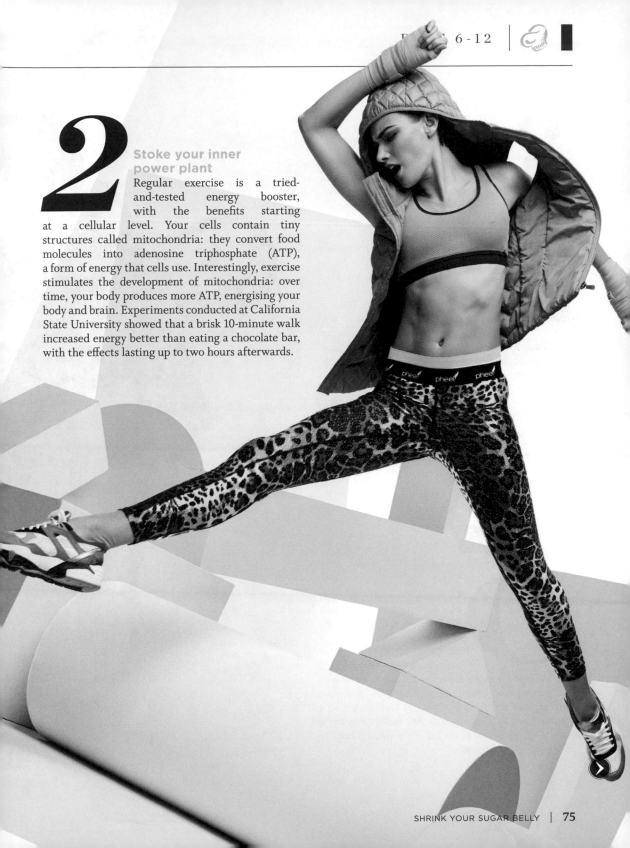

2

Stoke your inner power plant

Regular exercise is a tried-and-tested energy booster, with the benefits starting at a cellular level. Your cells contain tiny structures called mitochondria: they convert food molecules into adenosine triphosphate (ATP), a form of energy that cells use. Interestingly, exercise stimulates the development of mitochondria: over time, your body produces more ATP, energising your body and brain. Experiments conducted at California State University showed that a brisk 10-minute walk increased energy better than eating a chocolate bar, with the effects lasting up to two hours afterwards.

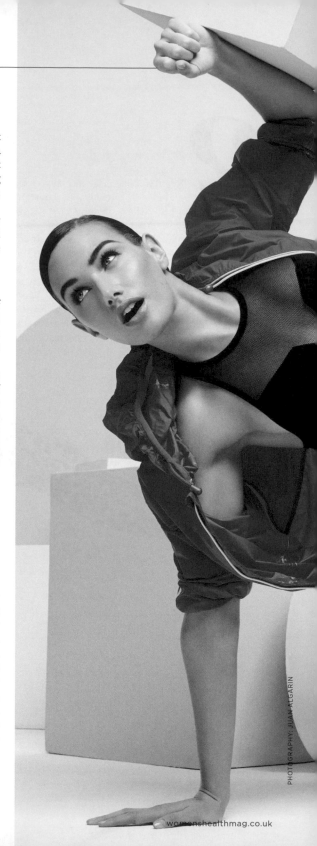

3 Take flight

If you're low on energy, you might want to head straight for the lift. But for a dose of instant pep, take the stairs – it will get your heart pumping, allowing oxygen-rich blood to surge through your entire body, including your brain.

So if your eyelids start to droop, get up and over to the stairs; climb a flight as quickly as you can and walk at a normal pace on the way down. Do this one more time and prepare to feel re-energised.

4 Take a break for tea

Tea's ability to deliver a relaxed state of alertness may be due to the amino acid L-theanine. Research indicates that tea's combination of caffeine and L-theanine delivers the same amount of energy as caffeine alone – but without the jitters.

One study examined the effects of 50 milligrams of L-theanine, the amount found in two cups of tea. Researchers gave 16 volunteers EEGs as they relaxed with their eyes closed. Compared with 19 other people who did not receive L-theanine, the participants who consumed this amino acid showed increased alpha-wave activity, indicating a relaxed but alert mental state. Get brewing.

5 Rejuvenate with ginseng

Exploit ginseng, another herb known for its energising qualities. In a 12-week study of 501 men and women, a group of participants given a multivitamin supplement that included ginseng reported having more energy and greater wellbeing than a group that received a ginseng-free supplement. Try 200 milligrams of a standardised extract taken as 100 milligrams twice daily. And stick with brands that are standardised to four per cent ginsenosides.

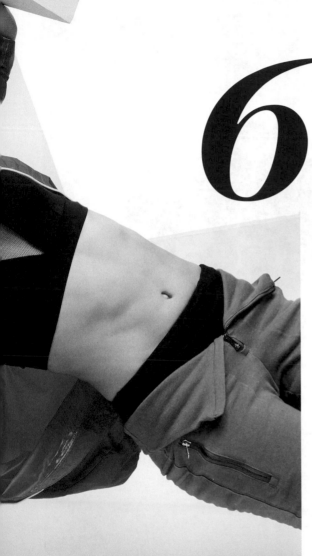

A brisk 10-minute walk was found to have increased energy better than eating a bar of chocolate

6 Step outside the box

The 'box' in this case is the four walls of your office or house: a series of studies found that spending just 20 minutes outside in nature can invigorate you. Researchers conducted separate experiments of 537 college students. In one experiment, students were led on a walk either indoors or outside along a tree-lined river path. In another, they looked at photos of buildings or landscapes. Other experiments had the students keep diaries in which they tracked their moods and energy levels throughout the day.

The results? The students consistently felt more energetic in natural settings or by imagining themselves in those surroundings.

7 Breathe in some energy

A simple yoga breathing exercise can clear your mind and raise your energy in minutes. It's called bhastrika, which translates as "bellows breath". Here's how to do it...

Sit comfortably. Relax your shoulders and take deep breaths. Begin to inhale and exhale rapidly through your nose, keeping your mouth closed but relaxed. Your breaths in and out should be equal in duration but as short as possible. Don't worry about this being noisy – it's supposed to be!

Try three in-and-out breath cycles per second. This will produce a quick movement of the diaphragm, suggesting a bellows. Breathe normally after each cycle. Do this for 15 seconds or less on your first try.

Each time you practice, increase your time by five seconds or so, until you reach a full minute. If you feel light-headed, stop for a minute, then start again with a little less force behind your breathing.

One more thing: don't try bellows breathing before bed, as it can easily keep you from falling asleep!

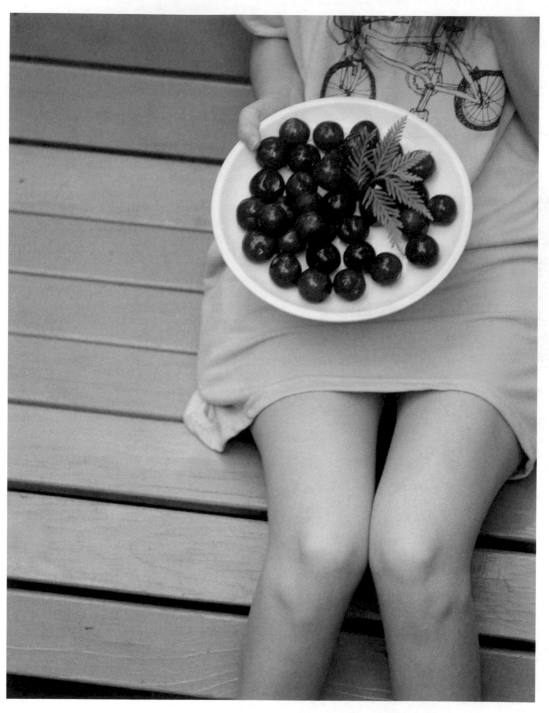

4

DAYS
13-20

+ NATURALLY SWEET + COMPLETELY SATISFYING +

Congratulations – you've made it this far without sugar. You should be feeling more energetic now your body's letting go of its attachment to the sweet stuff. And did we mention your skin might be glowing just a little? You've earned another reward; a little dose of sweetness. It's time to make friends with fruit again

84 Breakfasts
Even more of the protein-packed breakfasts that you've come to rely on – now with added fruit to brighten up your morning!

88 Main Meals
Mix it up! Even more energy and flavour-packed dishes that will make your taste buds happy without spiking your blood sugar.

92 Snacks
Blow your snacking horizons wide open by adding fruit, and learn how to make your own combinations with our handy, healthy treats grid.

98 Sugar-Belly Rules
Eating these delicious meals won't be a problem – but steering clear of additional treats might be. Here's how to stay on track to success.

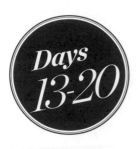

Days 13-20

PHASE 2
RETURN OF NATURE'S
ORIGINAL DESSERT

Trust us, after seven long days without any sugar, your brain's reward centre will experience that first bite of juicy pear, luscious grape or crunchy apple as an explosion of sweetness – a full-on parade of flavour marching across your taste buds. The part of your appetite that previously begged you for doughnuts will be just as satisfied with this phase's delectable, fruit-filled menu.

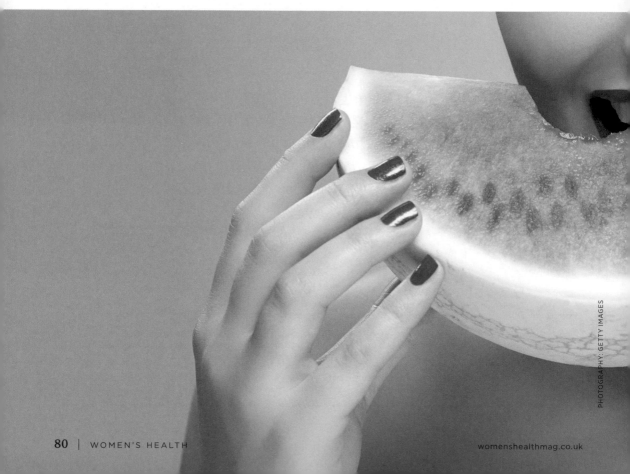

PHOTOGRAPHY: GETTY IMAGES

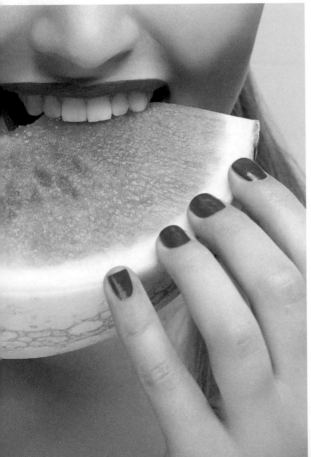

So why does fruit get a pass in your new phase? Simple – it's packed with fibre and nutrients, and it doesn't contain any added sugar. Now, you're currently working towards a goal of six teaspoons of added sugar a day, but not yet – it has to be done gradually. We've eliminated it on days 6–12 because a sugar-loaded palate will have been so over-sugared that it's lost the ability to really taste and appreciate the sweetness in fruit. Eliminating it for those seven days has helped to reset the way your taste buds and brain react to sugar stimuli.

We're not saying that fruit doesn't have sugar, or that the sugar isn't more or less chemically the same as the stuff found on top of your cereal or stirred into your tea (table sugar and the sugar in fruit have approximately the same proportion of fructose and glucose). But fruit has less of it, and the body has a harder time extracting the sugar from a piece of fruit than it does from a sweet. That's because fruit is packed with fibre, which slows the breakdown of the food in your digestive system, leading to a far more gradual release of sugar into your body – sparing you from the heady sugar spikes that used to send you reeling.

DAYS 13–20 **What to do**

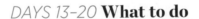

Have breakfast every morning. Just as you did in Phase 1, you'll start the day with a protein-packed meal to keep your appetite and blood sugar on an even keel. In this phase, you'll find some terrific fruit options. When fruit is paired with protein and fat, it's even more satisfying.

Feel free to mix and match the lunch and dinner options. You can also keep eating any of the Phase 1 meals, but we've added some quick and easy meals to this phase to keep it varied. Just like the Phase 1 meals, these are centred on fresh, whole foods – grains, vegetables, low-fat dairy and lean protein.

Have one serving of a processed wholegrain product, if you like. Ideally, all of your grain intake would be from whole unprocessed grains because once they're pulverised into flour and restructured into cereal, bread, or noodles – they get digested

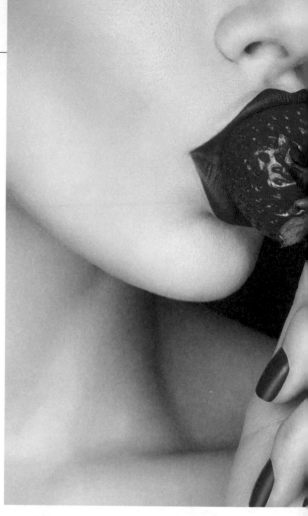

almost as quickly as sugar. But we all live in the real world, when a bowl of cold cereal makes for a quick breakfast, a bowl of pasta is calling your name, or you want the convenience of a sandwich. That's why we've brought back processed whole grain products in this phase, but just once a day. A note about bread: it can be tough to track down a commercial one that doesn't contain added sugar, so the bread we use on this phase comes in the form of tortillas and pittas, which tend to have about one gram or less. If you choose to eat one of our wrap or burrito options, you'd be taking in a minuscule amount of added sugar. If you opt for

Q: CAN I SWAP DRIED FRUIT OR FRUIT JUICE FOR FRESH FRUIT?

A: Dried fruit has all the fibre, nutrients and sugar of fresh, but concentrated into a smaller portion. For instance, a handful of fresh apricot halves has 37 calories and seven grams of sugar. A handful of dried apricot halves supply 157 calories and 35 grams of sugar. Rather than snacking on it, think of it as an added sugar, like honey or maple syrup, and use it as an ingredient in recipes to enhance the flavour. (Some dried fruit, like cranberries and tart cherries, are sweetened with sugar.) As such, the meals in this phase don't contain any dried fruit. Once your eating plan is over, you can reintroduce it in your new, healthier, sugar-smart recipes.

As for fruit juice, step away! If your goal is to shrink your sugar belly, it's best to satisfy your sweet tooth with fruit. Fruit juice has more sugar than fruit, and even though that sugar is still natural, it contributes calories. For instance, a regular glass of orange juice has 112 calories, 21 grams of sugar, and 0.5 grams of fibre. A medium orange has 69 calories, 12 grams of sugar, and three grams of fibre. The juice will be converted into blood sugar more quickly than the orange will. Moreover, calories that you drink simply don't fill you up. That's because liquids don't trigger your satiety mechanism the same way whole foods do, and juice doesn't have the critical fibre component that whole fruit offers.

cereal, pick one with zero grams of sugar and three or more grams of fibre per serving.

Have fruit up to three times a day. For all its nutritious goodness, fruit's sugar content means it's higher in calories than vegetables. So to keep your weight in check, you don't want to go overboard on the fruit. Whether you snack on it, serve it for dessert or eat it as part of a meal, you can have fruit as long as you don't eat more than three servings per day. (A serving is a selection of sliced fruit or one medium piece of whole fruit.) If strong sugar cravings have been an issue in the past, you may want to head for low-sugar fruits more often; it's best to play safe.

Don't forget to snack! Eating every few hours is just as important in this phase as it was in the last one. You'll still be eating one 100-calorie and one

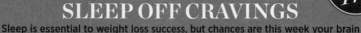

SLEEP OFF CRAVINGS

Sleep is essential to weight loss success, but chances are this week your brain will be nagging you to raid the fridge under cover of darkness – leaving you frazzled for the next day and much more likely to give in to sugar temptation. A small Harvard study using yoga breathing techniques to treat anxiety-based insomnia found that all volunteers reported better quality and quantity of sleep. To get the best possible, try a breathing technique called '4-7-8 breathing'. With your tongue resting on the roof of your mouth, just behind your upper teeth, exhale completely. Close your mouth then inhale through your nose for four counts. Hold your breath for seven counts, then exhale while counting to eight in your head. Repeat this three more times.

fighting, skin-boosting nutrients like antioxidants and phytochemicals. The real difference between types lies in their colours, which are linked to different nutritional goodies. The more shades you choose, the more health benefits you'll reap.

GET GRILLING

To turn fruit from a snack to a proper dessert, you've got to try grilling it, at least once. Grilling fruit causes its sugars to caramelise, creating a unique, smokey flavour that's perfect for a side dish or dessert that tastes decadent.

You can grill any fruit large and firm enough to take the heat — apples, pears, pineapple, peaches, oranges, even strawberries — if you put them on skewers. If you want to try grilling smaller fruits, like grapes or blueberries, use a pan to hold them above the flames or coals.

To prevent sticking, brush the fruit on both sides with about a teaspoon of olive oil. Most fruits need only three or four minutes of grilling on each side. Grill over a medium-low heat and don't walk away while it's cooking. When it's done, slide it onto a plate, top with a dollop of Greek yoghurt, ricotta or cottage cheese (trust us, it can work!) and dust with cinnamon.

150-calorie snack per day at the times of your choosing. And while you can have a juicy piece of fruit, we suggest that you pair it with protein or a fat in order to control your blood-sugar response and satisfy your appetite even more. Check out the chart on page 94 for some ideas.

Avoid the following foods: white flour and products made with it, white rice, fruit juice, and sugar in any of its many forms (including the table sugar you might add to foods; honey, agave and maple syrup).

EAT THE SPECTRUM

Think of fruits as crayons. You wouldn't use just two colours, right? You want the whole box to pick from. It's the same with fruit. All fruit contains fibre, vitamins, minerals and various disease-

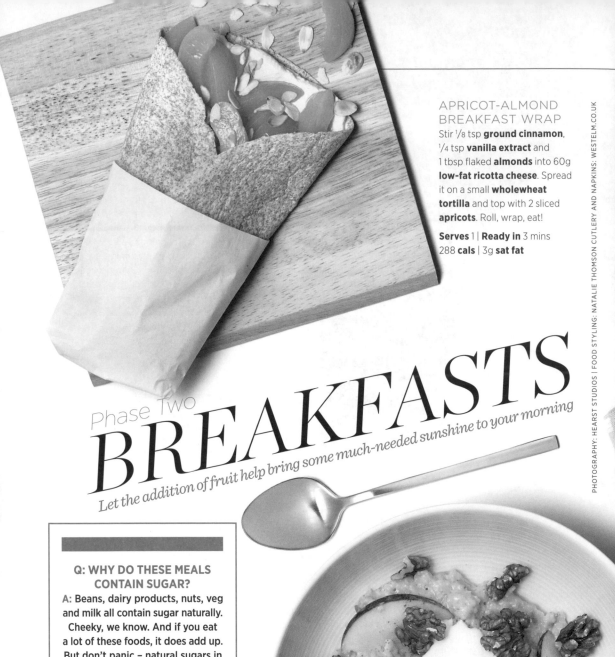

PHOTOGRAPHY: HEARST STUDIOS | FOOD STYLING: NATALIE THOMSON CUTLERY AND NAPKINS: WESTELM.CO.UK

APRICOT-ALMOND BREAKFAST WRAP

Stir $1/8$ tsp **ground cinnamon**, $1/4$ tsp **vanilla extract** and 1 tbsp flaked **almonds** into 60g **low-fat ricotta cheese**. Spread it on a small **wholewheat tortilla** and top with 2 sliced **apricots**. Roll, wrap, eat!

Serves 1 | **Ready in** 3 mins
288 **cals** | 3g **sat fat**

Phase Two
BREAKFASTS

Let the addition of fruit help bring some much-needed sunshine to your morning

Q: WHY DO THESE MEALS CONTAIN SUGAR?

A: Beans, dairy products, nuts, veg and milk all contain sugar naturally. Cheeky, we know. And if you eat a lot of these foods, it does add up. But don't panic – natural sugars in foods are not 'added sugar' (ie: the kind you need to worry about). And these recipes will give you the amount of natural sugar you need so you can get a sense of which foods contain sugar naturally (and how much of it) to help you make healthy food choices.

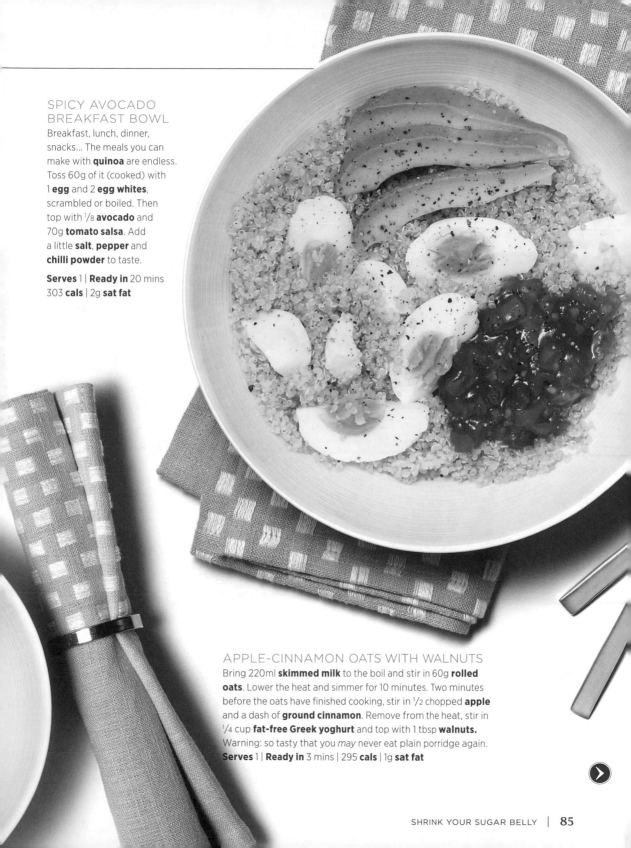

SPICY AVOCADO BREAKFAST BOWL

Breakfast, lunch, dinner, snacks... The meals you can make with **quinoa** are endless. Toss 60g of it (cooked) with 1 **egg** and 2 **egg whites**, scrambled or boiled. Then top with 1/8 **avocado** and 70g **tomato salsa**. Add a little **salt**, **pepper** and **chilli powder** to taste.

Serves 1 | **Ready in** 20 mins
303 **cals** | 2g **sat fat**

APPLE-CINNAMON OATS WITH WALNUTS

Bring 220ml **skimmed milk** to the boil and stir in 60g **rolled oats**. Lower the heat and simmer for 10 minutes. Two minutes before the oats have finished cooking, stir in 1/2 chopped **apple** and a dash of **ground cinnamon**. Remove from the heat, stir in 1/4 cup **fat-free Greek yoghurt** and top with 1 tbsp **walnuts.** Warning: so tasty that you *may* never eat plain porridge again.
Serves 1 | **Ready in** 3 mins | 295 **cals** | 1g **sat fat**

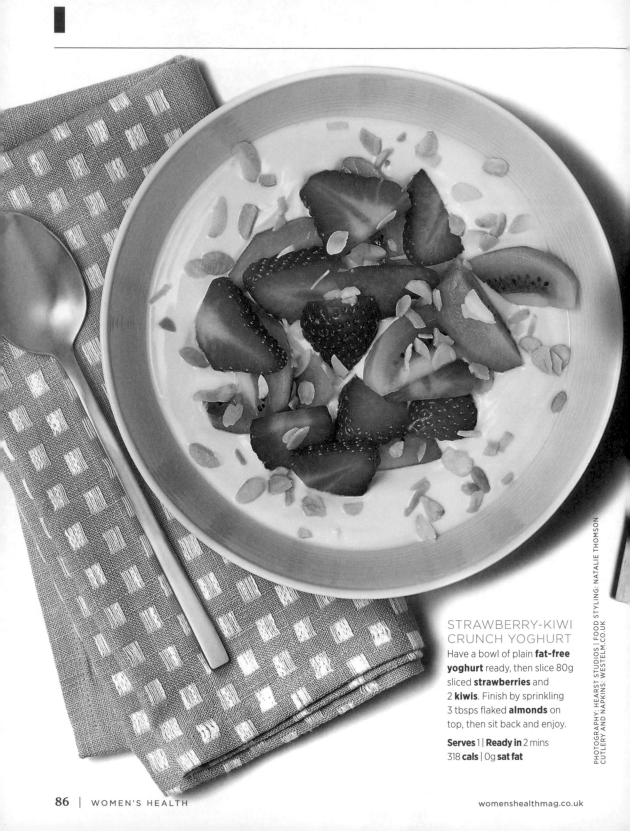

STRAWBERRY-KIWI CRUNCH YOGHURT

Have a bowl of plain **fat-free yoghurt** ready, then slice 80g sliced **strawberries** and 2 **kiwis**. Finish by sprinkling 3 tbsps flaked **almonds** on top, then sit back and enjoy.

Serves 1 | **Ready in** 2 mins
318 **cals** | 0g **sat fat**

PHOTOGRAPHY: HEARST STUDIOS | FOOD STYLING: NATALIE THOMSON
CUTLERY AND NAPKINS: WESTELM.CO.UK

Q: CAN I HAVE A BEER OR A GLASS OF WINE?
A: Try not to drink alcohol during the eating plan because it adds extra calories. But if, during Phase 2 and beyond, you decide to have a cheeky drink, stick to half a pint of beer, a small glass of wine or one shot of spirits – count it as your 100-calorie snack for that day. Limit your drinks to two per week.

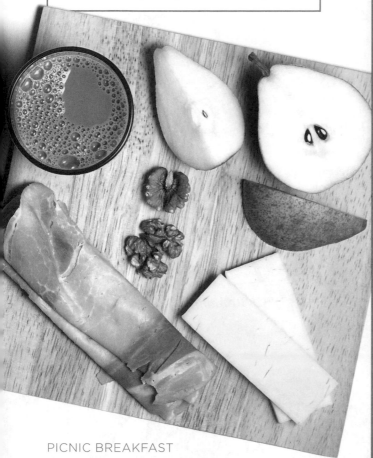

PICNIC BREAKFAST

This fuss-free selection works come rain or shine. Place 30g **low-fat Cheddar cheese**, a slice of **deli ham**, 2 **walnut halves** and 1 **pear** on a plate or chopping board. Wash down with a small **latte**. (Sunglasses are optional.)

Serves 1 | **Ready in** 2 mins | 297 **cals** | 4g **sat fat**

RUN RINGS AROUND TEMPTATION

Are everyday life hassles what make you reach for sugar? Here's how to see off your stress without pounding a jumbo bag of Tangfastics

Circle breathing is a simple way to relieve stress fast, and you can do it anywhere, at any time. When you're anxious, off centre, or feel like you'll explode, do a round of circle breathing – five to 10 breaths should do it. During Days 6-12, aim to use this exercise five or more times a day, to help your body and mind form a strong, positive habit. What's more, according to a recent study in the *Journal of Alternative and Complementary Medicine*, relaxation breathing after meals helps prevent glucose spikes.

1 Inhale and stretch your arms over your head. Exhale, sighing as you lower them. Relax and keep your arms lowered for the rest of the exercise.

2 Now imagine that you're inhaling a stream of peaceful energy into a spot about a few inches below your navel.

3 Continue inhaling, imagining the energy travelling to the base of your spine, then imagine it travelling up your back to the top of your head.

4 Exhale, and mentally follow that breath back down the front of your body to the point below your navel where you'll begin the next inhale. Your breath has now made a full circle – up the back of your body, down the front and back to the starting place below your navel.

5 Do five to 10 circle breaths. You can also use circle breaths for a longer period as a form of meditation.

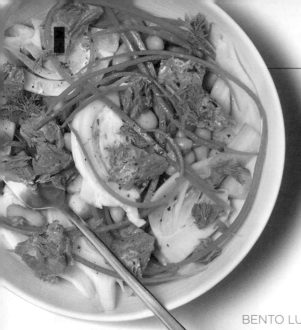

FENNEL COLESLAW WITH SALMON AND WHITE BEANS

Whisk 1 tbsp **apple cider vinegar**, 2 tsps **olive oil**, ½ tsp **dried oregano** and ½ tsp **Dijon mustard** to make a dressing for the 'slaw. Then toss 90g thinly sliced **fennel bulb**, 30g shredded **carrot**, 30g thinly sliced **cucumber**, 250g tinned **white beans** (rinsed and drained) into a bowl, mix up well and drizzle with the **dressing**. Gently stir in 80g tinned **salmon**, then tuck in!

Serves 1 | **Ready in** 15 mins | 463 **cals** | 2g **sat fat**

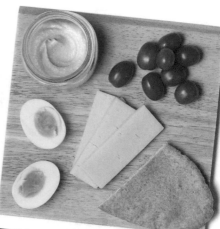

BENTO LUNCHBOX

For a portable, protein-packed meal, have a hard-boiled **egg** with 30g **Cheddar cheese**, 150g **cherry tomatoes**, 60g **houmous** and half of a **wholewheat pitta**.

Serves 1 | **Ready in** 7 mins
412 **cals** | 8g **sat fat**

Phase Two
MAIN MEALS

Add these new options to existing Phase 1 meals on your menu

SPINACH AND BULGUR SALAD, TOPPED WITH GRAPEFRUIT AND GRILLED CHICKEN

With a fork, whisk 1 tsp **apple cider vinegar**, 2 tsps **olive oil**, ¼ tsp **dried thyme** and ¼ tsp **crushed garlic** until it's mixed up well. Set your dressing aside, then layer up your salad in a bowl: 50g **baby spinach** and 100g cooked **bulgur**. Top with 150g **grapefruit** segments and 85g sliced **grilled chicken**.

Serves 1 | **Ready in** 15 mins
388 **cals** | 2g **sat fat**

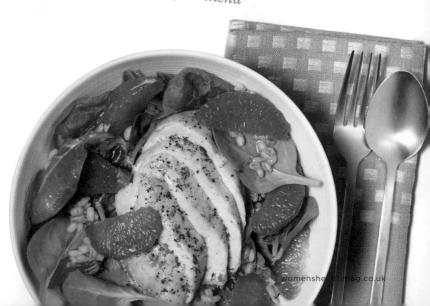

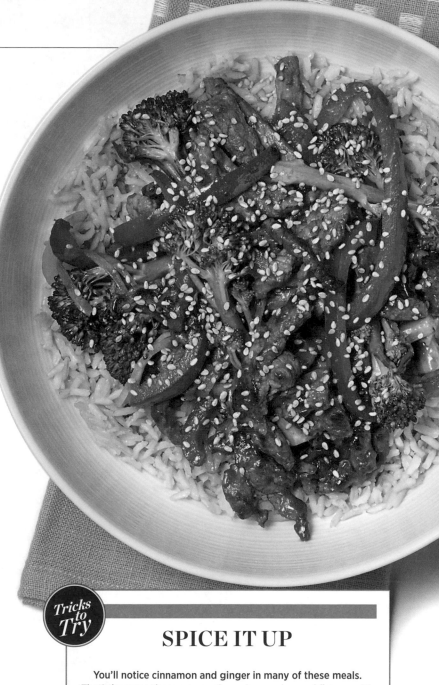

TERIYAKI BEEF WITH BROCCOLI

* 70ml **teriyaki sauce**
* 70ml **soy sauce**
* 340g **skirt steak**, sliced into thin strips across the grain
* 450ml **chicken stock**
* 230g **brown rice**
* 2 tsps **canola oil**
* ½ **onion**, sliced
* 1 **red pepper**, sliced
* 300g **broccoli florets**
* 2 tsps **cornflour**
* ¼ tsp **red pepper flakes**
* 2 tbsps **toasted sesame seeds**

1/ In a large bowl, pour the teriyaki sauce over the beef. Cover with cling film and put it in the fridge for 1-10 hours.
2/ In a saucepan, bring the stock and rice to a boil, then simmer, covered, for 40 minutes or until all the water is absorbed.
3/ Heat the oil in a wok and cook the onion, pepper and broccoli for 5 minutes. Transfer to a separate bowl.
4/ Drain the beef – but hold on to the excess teriyaki sauce! Dip the meat in the cornflour and whack it in the wok, over a high heat, for 3 minutes. Then add the vegetables, pepper flakes and leftover teriyaki sauce to the mix and cook for another 2 minutes.
5/ Serve the teriyaki meat and veg over the rice and sprinkle with the sesame seeds. Who needs a takeaway?

Serves 4 | **Ready in** 15 + 60 mins
462 **cals** | 6g **sat fat**

PHOTOGRAPHY: HEARST STUDIOS | FOOD STYLING: NATALIE THOMSON CUTLERY AND NAPKINS: WESTELM.CO.UK

Tricks to Try

SPICE IT UP

You'll notice cinnamon and ginger in many of these meals. That's because these warm spices give you bags of flavour with none of the sugar. Cinnamon in particular has been found to help lower blood sugar, which impacts on your body's ability to burn fat. Sprinkle it on yoghurt, popcorn, ricotta – any bland food that's crying out for some fat-burning flavour!

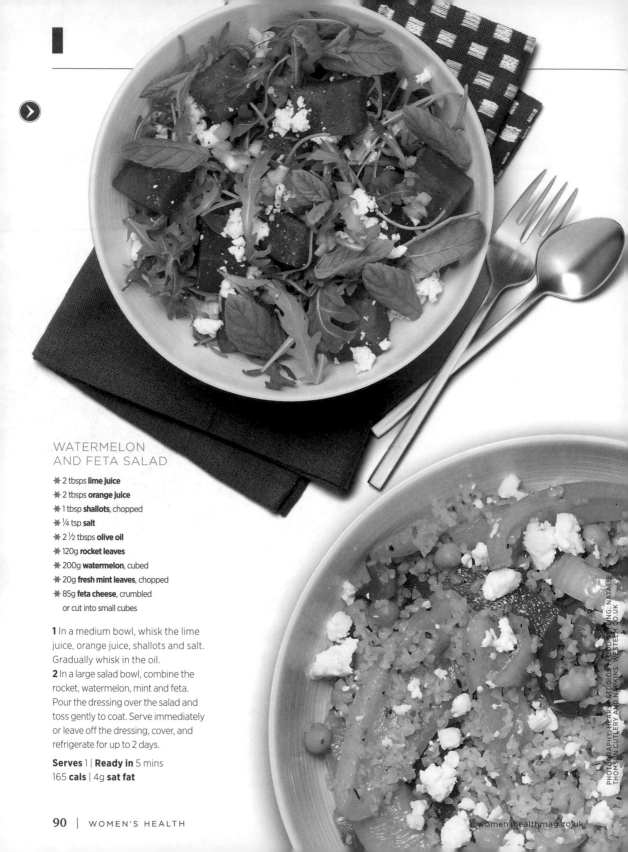

WATERMELON AND FETA SALAD

- ✳ 2 tbsps **lime juice**
- ✳ 2 tbsps **orange juice**
- ✳ 1 tbsp **shallots**, chopped
- ✳ ¼ tsp **salt**
- ✳ 2 ½ tbsps **olive oil**
- ✳ 120g **rocket leaves**
- ✳ 200g **watermelon**, cubed
- ✳ 20g **fresh mint leaves**, chopped
- ✳ 85g **feta cheese**, crumbled
  or cut into small cubes

1 In a medium bowl, whisk the lime juice, orange juice, shallots and salt. Gradually whisk in the oil.
2 In a large salad bowl, combine the rocket, watermelon, mint and feta. Pour the dressing over the salad and toss gently to coat. Serve immediately or leave off the dressing, cover, and refrigerate for up to 2 days.

Serves 1 | **Ready in** 5 mins
165 **cals** | 4g **sat fat**

PHOTOGRAPHY: HEARST STUDIOS. FOOD STYLING: NATALIE THOMSON. CUTLERY AND NAPKINS: WESTELM.CO.UK

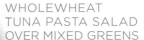

WHOLEWHEAT TUNA PASTA SALAD OVER MIXED GREENS

You know what to do: make your dressing by whisking 1 tbsp **lemon juice**, 2 tsps **olive oil**, ¼ tsp **dried basil** and ¼ tsp **crushed garlic**. In a bowl, put 140g of cooked **wholewheat spiral pasta**, 3 tbsps **black olives** and half of a 140g tinned, drained **water-packed tuna**. Serve over 30g **mixed leaves** and top with your dressing. Done.

Serves 1 | **Ready in** 7 mins
396 **cals** | 2g **sat fat**

ROASTED VEGETABLE, BULGUR AND CHICKPEA SALAD WITH FETA DRESSING

- ✳ 500ml **low-salt vegetable stock**
- ✳ 182g **dry bulgur wheat**
- ✳ 4 **peppers**, sliced
- ✳ 1 **onion**, diced
- ✳ 6 tbsps **olive oil**
- ✳ 1 (400g) tin **chickpeas** drained
- ✳ 5 tbsps **red wine vinegar**
- ✳ 3 tbsps **lemon juice**
- ✳ 2 tsps **crushed garlic**
- ✳ 1 tsp **dried oregano**
- ✳ 120g **crumbled feta cheese**

1/ Pre-heat the oven to 200°C.
2/ In a saucepan, bring the broth to a boil before adding the bulgur. Cover the pot until the broth begins to boil, then remove the saucepan from the heat. Allow the cooked bulgur to sit for 20 minutes.
3/ On a baking tray, place the peppers and onion with 4 tsps of the oil. Bake for 10 minutes, then flip over peppers and onion, and add the chickpeas to the tray.

4/ Cook for another 10 minutes, or until the onion is golden and both onion and peppers are soft.
5/ In a small bowl, whisk together the vinegar, lemon juice, garlic, oregano, feta and the remaining 4 teaspoons oil. Toss the chickpea and veg mixture with the bulgur and drizzle with the dressing.

Serves 461 | **Ready in** 40 mins
461 **cals** | 5g **sat fat**

EAT WITH AWARENESS

Cut unwanted calories when you master the art of mindful eating

When you eat in a mindful manner, you're fully aware of the flavours, textures and aromas of every bite. You'll find you enjoy your food more and that you're easily satiated.

Try mindful eating at your next meal. It's worth doing the first few times alone and after a while, you should feel comfortable eating mindfully when dining with others.

1 Sit at the table, with your plate in front of you. Before you pick up your fork, take a couple of deep breaths to allow your body and mind to settle.

2 Look at your food. The Vietnamese Buddhist monk Thich Nhat Hanh developed an exercise in which the participant considers the journey of the food to the person eating it. They would imagine all of the phases an orange has passed through to grow and travel to them, and be grateful to the tree and sun for growing it.

3 Take a bite, taking time to observe your fork rising to your mouth. Place it on your tongue and chew, tuning in to its flavour, temperature and texture.

4 Chew each bite for at least 20 seconds. By turning your focus inward and concentrating on the taste and smell, eating can feel brand new.

5 Notice your thoughts and feelings. Do you like what you're eating? Do you wish it was sweeter or saltier? Are you still hungry or getting full?

6 As you finish, take a few deep breaths. Remind yourself of how the plate looked when it was full and how it looks now.

YOGHURT-COVERED BLUEBERRIES

✳ 170g fat-free plain **Greek yoghurt** ✳ 1 teaspoon **vanilla extract**
✳ 200g **fresh blueberries**

1/ Cover a large baking tray with foil or parchment paper.
2/ In a blender, zap the yoghurt, vanilla extract and 70g of the blueberries.
3/ Using a toothpick or your fingers, dip and coat the remaining blueberries into the yoghurt mixture.
4/ Place each blueberry on the baking tray and freeze for an hour. And if you don't fancy snacking on them *right* now, you can freeze them in an airtight container for up to a week.
Serves 1 | **Ready in** 75 mins
154 **cals** | 3g **sat fat**

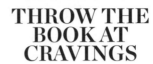

THROW THE BOOK AT CRAVINGS

A study by the University of Sussex found reading can slash stress by 68 per cent. Researchers also discovered that sipping a cup of tea worked too (54 per cent). Pick a quiet spot where you won't be interrupted and sip on a calming tea, such as camomile, while you turn the pages. (Maybe give *Charlie and the Chocolate Factory* a miss, though.)

Tricks to Try

Phase Two
SNACKS
Fill your week with these fruity filler-uppers

CREAMY DARK CHOCOLATE– BANANA-COCONUT PUDDING

✴ 3 ripe **bananas** ✴ 15g **unsweetened cocoa powder** ✴ 240g plain fat-free **Greek yoghurt** ✴ 1 tsp **vanilla extract** ✴ 3 tbsp **unsweetened coconut flakes**

1/ Did someone say chocolate? Quick – mash the bananas in a bowl until smooth and creamy.
2/ Add the cocoa powder, yoghurt, vanilla and 1 tbsp of the coconut to the bananas. Using a fork, stir vigorously for 3 minutes, or until all of the ingredients are well combined.

3/ Divide the pudding into four small bowls or ramekins. Sprinkle each one with the remaining coconut flakes. Refrigerate for 30 minutes and serve chilled. Cool stuff.

Serves 2 | **Ready in** 40 mins
154 **cals** | 3g **sat fat**

BUILD YOUR OWN PHASE 2 SNACK

When cravings come to call, there are literally thousands of options available to you that don't involve added sugar. Simply choose one protein source from the grid below, then pair it with the fruit portion of your choice. Hey presto – you've got yourself a tummy-filling, energy-boosting, skin-glowing taste explosion on your hands. Careful now.

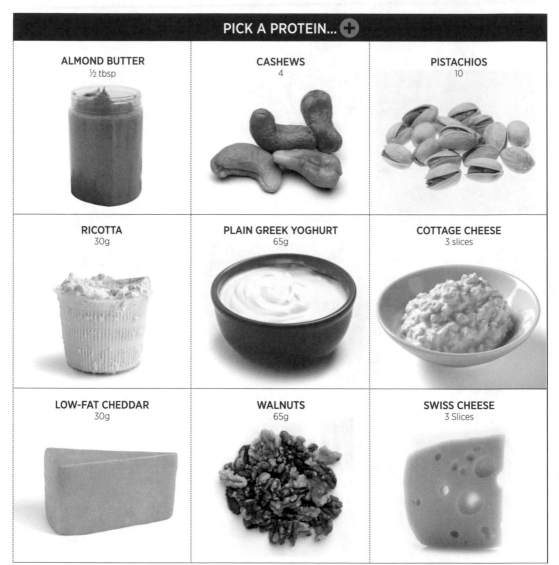

PICK A PROTEIN... +

ALMOND BUTTER
½ tbsp

CASHEWS
4

PISTACHIOS
10

RICOTTA
30g

PLAIN GREEK YOGHURT
65g

COTTAGE CHEESE
3 slices

LOW-FAT CHEDDAR
30g

WALNUTS
65g

SWISS CHEESE
3 Slices

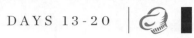
⊕ ...THEN ADD SOME FRUIT

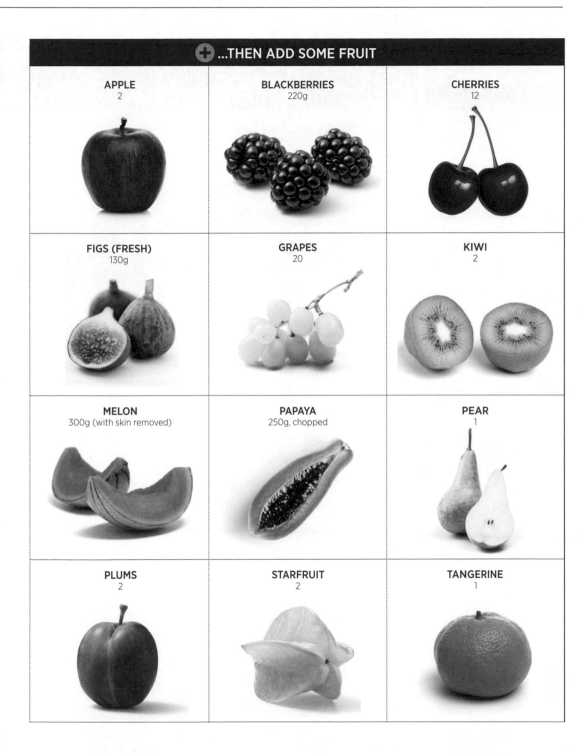

APPLE 2	BLACKBERRIES 220g	CHERRIES 12
FIGS (FRESH) 130g	GRAPES 20	KIWI 2
MELON 300g (with skin removed)	PAPAYA 250g, chopped	PEAR 1
PLUMS 2	STARFRUIT 2	TANGERINE 1

YOUR PHASE 2 EATING LOG

BREAKFAST	SNACK	LUNCH	SNACK
Day 1			
Day 2			
Day 3			
Day 4			
Day 5			
Day 6			
Day 7			
Day 8			

DINNER	WORKOUT	TIPS I TRIED	HOW I FEEL

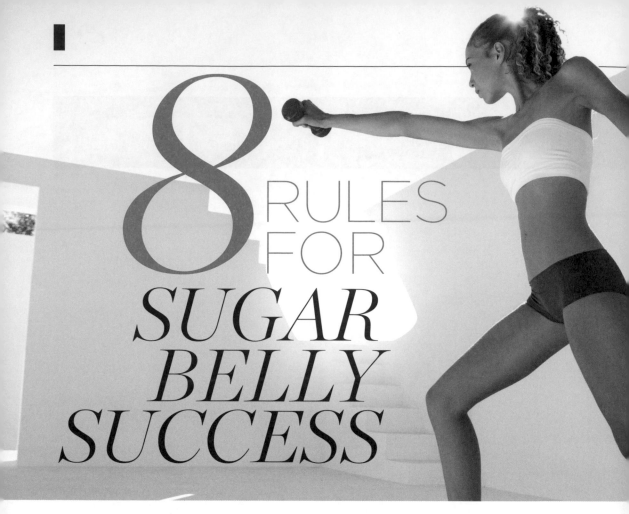

8 RULES FOR SUGAR BELLY SUCCESS

If you follow the 20-day *Shrink Your Sugar Belly* plan to the very letter, you'll find that the meals, snacks, tips and strategies will cut the extra wadding from your waist and transform your body's ability to withstand temptation. But bad habits are always initially hard to break, which is why we've put together some next-level mind, body and stomach tricks to help keep you on track. Commit to them before you start, and the results will delight you.

Here's a snapshot from your future: you've shrunk your sugar belly, but you've also accomplished so much more. The afternoon desk-slump, only banished by a trip to the bakery, no longer affects your productivity. The creases around your eyes and mouth somehow seem less... well, *creased.* You're healthy, calm and no longer troubled by cravings.

But the best bit? You're still treating yourself – when it matters. You've crushed your dependence on sugar but reclaimed the pleasure, and these eight guidelines have made it all possible. Make sure they go from this page into your head; write them out as a list and keep them somewhere visible. And, once your 20 days are up, stick to them for as long as you want.

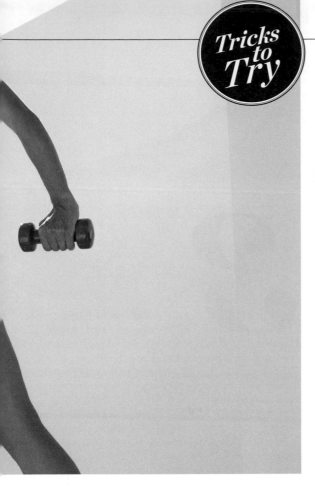

Tricks to Try

1 Begin your day with breakfast, and pack it with protein

You've probably heard this a million times, but breakfast really is the most important meal of the day, especially if you're looking to slim down. In fact, eating a morning meal is a common habit among people who have lost weight and kept it off. Breakfast skippers are four and a half times more likely to be obese than breakfast eaters, a study in the *American Journal of Epidemiology* showed. Another study from the Harvard Medical School in Boston, Massachusetts found that eating breakfast led to better blood-sugar control, cutting in half the odds of having the high-glucose levels that can lead to higher levels of fat being stored on your body.

What you eat is important, though. Start your day with cold cereal (even wholegrain), a bagel, or some fruit and chances are you will be ravenous in just a few hours. Why? Those meals are primarily carbohydrates – and quickly digested ones at that. Glucose levels spike and insulin is released, glucose levels plummet and you're left scrounging for a snack. And it's not likely it'll be something healthy.

The antidote: pump up the protein. It slows digestion and research shows that calorie for calorie, protein is more filling than carbohydrates or fat. Researchers at Saint Louis University found that overweight women naturally took in about 160 fewer calories at lunch when they ate protein-packed eggs in the morning instead of a bagel.

Other research shows that protein in the morning makes it difficult for sugar cravings to take hold later on. Researchers at the University of Missouri had 20 overweight young women who routinely skipped breakfast either eat one of two morning meals, cereal or eggs and beef, or no breakfast at all for seven days. On that last day, the women took part in a 10-hour test that included an all-you-can-eat dinner of microwave pizza, as well as unlimited evening snacks such as biscuits, cake, apple slices and yoghurt.

The results? The high-protein egg-beef group produced less of the hunger-stimulating hormone ghrelin and more of the fullness hormone PPY than those who ate cereal. MRI scans showed reduced activity in areas of the brain associated with cravings. The protein group reported a 30 per cent increase in feelings of fullness and consumed 170 fewer calories by the time they got to the evening snack.

Breakfasts on the *Shrink Your Sugar Belly* plan are hearty – around 300 calories, with at least 20 per cent coming from protein. Your breakfasts are stuffed with a yummy range of lean-protein dairy and nut goodies, from Greek yoghurt, eggs and low-fat cheese to peanut butter and quinoa.

If you can't stomach food too early in the morning, eat it by 10am and breakfast will still work hard on your behalf to help quell late-day cravings.

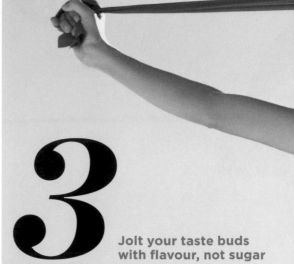

2 Never go hungry – simply eat five times a day

We told you why you shouldn't skip breakfast. Now we'll tell you why you shouldn't skip lunch, dinner or snacks, either.

We know – sometimes it's unavoidable. You're on a can't-miss deadline. Your dog is ill, and the vet appointment is at lunch. Or you're just honest-to-goodness not hungry, so you think that if you skip a meal that you don't want anyway, it will save you a few calories. But there's a danger in meal skipping – weight and sugar-belly peril. If you cut down on the amount of food you eat for an extended period of time, your body is going to slow things down to conserve its energy supply.

If you're looking to flatten your sugar belly, that 'starvation' response is the last thing you need. Meal skipping is also a guaranteed way to fire up sugar cravings. Skipping meals lowers blood-sugar levels and causes you to over-eat for the rest of the day to make up for missed calories.

However, we're predicting that you won't want to miss any meals or snacks while following the 20-day eating plan. Made with nourishing, delicious whole foods – such as wholegrains, beans, lean meats/poultry/fish, nuts, unsweetened low-fat dairy, eggs, and vegetables – they'll fill you up and give you the balance of lean protein, energising carbohydrates, and healthy fats to steady your blood sugar and insulin levels and extinguish cravings for sugar.

3 Jolt your taste buds with flavour, not sugar

What's the difference between the two? As delightful as sugar is, it always tastes the same, with variations on sweet and sickeningly sweet. On the other hand, flavour is diverse and surprising – if you expose your taste buds to those flavours.

If you've ever laid fresh sprigs of rosemary on chicken as it roasts, seeded a deliciously fragrant vanilla bean for a special dessert or topped a sliced tomato with basil leaves, you know how much flavour fresh herbs and spices can add to everyday fare.

And as you'll come to learn, sweet spices, such as cinnamon, can ease cravings for sugar. And when a dish calls for fresh herbs, do your best to use them. Leafy basil, coriander, parsley, mint, dill and thyme are far more flavourful than their dried counterparts. Don't forget other flavour boosters – balsamic vinegar, lemon and orange zest, roasted peppers, hot sauce, toasted nuts and home-made salsa, to name a few. One of the most effective is extra-virgin olive oil, giving a grassy, fruity flavour to salads, vegetables and soups; even a little drizzle gives an "I'm-feeling-full" sensation. Just getting a whiff reduced the number of calories people consumed at a meal and even improved their blood-sugar response, according to a study from the Munich-based German Research Center for Food Chemistry. Amazing!

As you move through the phases of the plan, identify which flavours thrill your tastebuds and commit to exploring the diverse array on offer to you – it might even help to start writing them down in

PHOTOGRAPHY: GETTY IMAGES

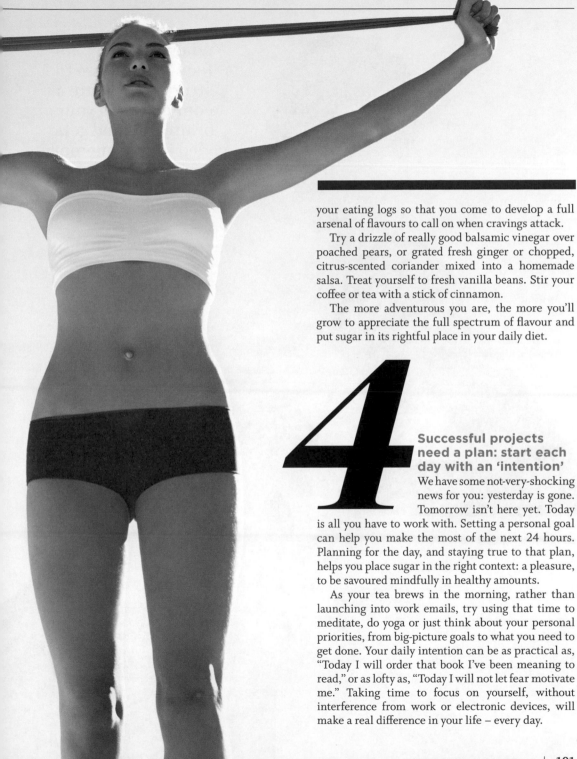

your eating logs so that you come to develop a full arsenal of flavours to call on when cravings attack.

Try a drizzle of really good balsamic vinegar over poached pears, or grated fresh ginger or chopped, citrus-scented coriander mixed into a homemade salsa. Treat yourself to fresh vanilla beans. Stir your coffee or tea with a stick of cinnamon.

The more adventurous you are, the more you'll grow to appreciate the full spectrum of flavour and put sugar in its rightful place in your daily diet.

4 Successful projects need a plan: start each day with an 'intention'

We have some not-very-shocking news for you: yesterday is gone. Tomorrow isn't here yet. Today is all you have to work with. Setting a personal goal can help you make the most of the next 24 hours. Planning for the day, and staying true to that plan, helps you place sugar in the right context: a pleasure, to be savoured mindfully in healthy amounts.

As your tea brews in the morning, rather than launching into work emails, try using that time to meditate, do yoga or just think about your personal priorities, from big-picture goals to what you need to get done. Your daily intention can be as practical as, "Today I will order that book I've been meaning to read," or as lofty as, "Today I will not let fear motivate me." Taking time to focus on yourself, without interference from work or electronic devices, will make a real difference in your life – every day.

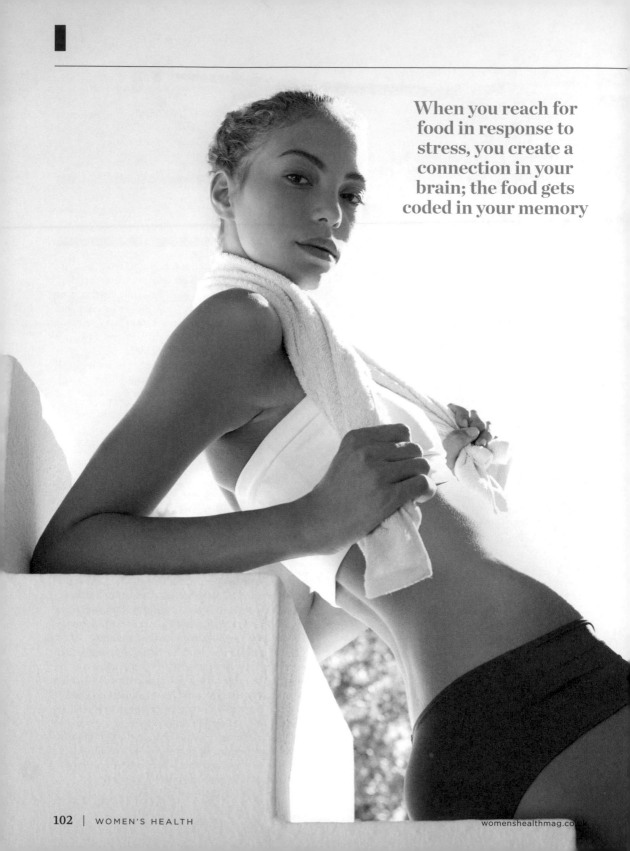

When you reach for food in response to stress, you create a connection in your brain; the food gets coded in your memory

5 Tone your belly by adding some joy to your life each day

We can almost hear you now: "With what time?" Well, maybe the time you spend complaining about traffic jams, the minutes grumbling about chaotic schedules and other common stresses you can't control. To lose weight and shrink your sugar belly, it's vital to commit to everyday rest and relaxation. Otherwise, chronic stress may eventually gain the upper hand and grind your physical and emotional wellbeing to dust.

Chronic stress – a daily assault of stress hormones from a demanding job or a life in turmoil – grinds away every cell in your body. That wear and tear comes at a price. Numerous emotional and physical disorders have been linked to stress, including depression, anxiety, heart attack, stroke, hypertension, digestive problems, even autoimmune diseases like rheumatoid arthritis.

You may also hit the chocolate and ice cream pretty hard. When you're stressed, your body releases the hormone cortisol, which signals your brain to seek rewards. Foods loaded with sugar and fat calm down that stress response by blunting this hormone. When you reach for food in response to stress, you inadvertently create a powerful connection in your brain. The food gets coded in your memory centre as a solution to an unpleasant experience or emotion. Face that same problem again and your brain will probably tell you, "Go and find some cupcakes!"

While you can't banish stress from your life completely, you can create an oasis of calm in your daily routine. Managing your stress requires that you find and maintain a balance between the stressful activities that drain you and the relaxing activities that refresh and renew your body and spirit. In each phase of the *Shrink Your Sugar Belly* plan, you'll discover stress-management techniques that you can build into your day. These simple but powerful strategies don't have to disrupt your busy schedule.

For example, if you like oranges, pick up a bottle of orange-scented aromatherapy oil or spray and treat yourself to a hit of 'sweet' without the sugar. In a study published in the *Journal of Alternative and Complementary Medicine,* participants who endured a stressful test felt much less anxious when they sniffed orange essential oil five minutes before the exam. Best of all, the effects followed them throughout the day.

Keeping a scented oil or spray at your desk can truly save the day. When you're in crunch time, pause and take a deep whiff. Wham! It's the modern-day equivalent of stopping to smell the roses. We've got lots more relaxation strategies like this in store. Small things can deliver pretty sweet rewards!

6 Sleep more to eat (and crave sugary treats) less

One important goal of the *Shrink Your Sugar Belly* plan is to restore metabolic harmony between the hormones ghrelin (an appetite trigger) and leptin (which signals satiety), along with insulin. When these hormones are working in harmony, the result is fewer cravings and less propensity to store fat.

But if you get less than the recommended seven to nine hours sleep a night, you may be undercutting this goal. In a University of Chicago study, a few sleepless nights were enough to drop levels of leptin by 18 per cent and boost levels of ghrelin by about 30 per cent. Those two changes alone caused appetites to kick into overdrive, and cravings for sugary foods like biscuits, buttered bread and cake jumped by 45 per cent. Not desirable.

Another reason to get to bed at a decent hour is that sleep deprivation may not only make sugary, fatty foods more appealing, it may also lower your ability to resist them, according to two small yet intriguing studies presented at a 2012 annual meeting of sleep researchers.

In one study of 25 men and women, researchers at Columbia University and Mount ´Sinai St Luke's/ Roosevelt Hospitals in New York used brain scans to compare activity in the brain's reward regions after five nights of either normal sleep (a restful nine hours) or restricted sleep (four hours). The scans were performed as the researchers showed their volunteers pictures of both healthy foods (items like fruit, vegetables and oatmeal) and unhealthy foods (chocolate, sweets and pizza). The reward regions were more active when the volunteers were sleep deprived than when they were well rested – especially when the sleepy subjects viewed the pictures of the sweets and pizza.

Worse, the parts of your brain that usually put the brakes on cravings aren't as active when you're tired, research conducted at the University of California in Berkeley found. Scientists had 16 people rate their desire for various foods – once after a night of normal sleep and once after 24 hours without sleep – as they administered brain scans.

The volunteers expressed a stronger preference for junk food when they were deprived of sleep. But the scans didn't just show more activity in reward regions. They also showed less activity in regions involved in decision making. So what is the upshot? When you're tired and fatigued, you are more likely to be drawn to sugary, fatty foods partly because your ability to process information and make sound decisions is impaired.

If there's anything humans should know how to do perfectly, it's sleep. However, our tech-heavy, stress-laden, long-commute lifestyles can make it hard to do what should come naturally (and for those with children, you can multiply the effects; but remember, sleep-training toddlers really works and only takes a few nights!). Throughout the plan we'll be offering simple ways to slide into the restful slumber you need for the best results and optimum wellbeing – each and every night – and wake up with new energy for your next day of sugar-busting eating.

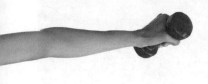

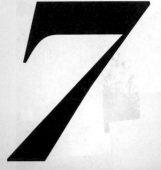

Now's the time to fix what's really bothering you

You certainly can't remember this, but from the moment you were born, you associated sugar with comfort. Newborn babies derive comfort from skin-to-skin contact, sucking, and their mother's milk, which is rich in lactose and naturally sweet. (Even if you were bottle-fed, you had the sweetness of lactose in your formula milk.) The link between comfort and sweet is primal – and persistent. The first step to breaking that emotional connection to sugar is to become aware of the feelings that drive you to it.

In each phase of the *Shrink Your Sugar Belly* plan you'll learn emotional coping strategies to help you ask just that. Whether or not to eat a biscuit isn't about need. It's about a decision. On the road to sugar freedom, making a conscious choice about sugar, regardless of how you feel, is an important milestone.

Exercise away your cravings

Exercise has a positive effect on appetite and blood-sugar metabolism, but it can be tough to fit a workout into a busy day. You need to create a workout that is convenient, pleasurable (nothing too sweaty or gruelling) and effective at helping to shrink a sugar belly. The workouts found in Chapter 5 of this book combine cardio exercise, strength training and yoga for an access-all-areas, three-pronged attack on blood sugar and cravings.

If you're plagued by strong sugar cravings, getting more active may help to de-activate them. According to a study published in *Applied Physiology, Nutrition, and Metabolism*, the more you sit, the greater your appetite – even if your body doesn't need the calories. Inactivity spurs secretion of ghrelin.

Moderate exercise also helps keep muscle cells sensitive to insulin. Even better, strength training builds muscle density – stronger muscles that use more glucose. And, like cardio, strength training aids weight loss.

Even if you don't want to follow the workouts supplied in this book, any physical activity that you actually enjoy will help get sugar off your brain – and belly. Brisk walking and t'ai chi both speed up metabolism as they quieten and divert the mind. City dwellers have plenty of opportunities to get the heart pumping: take the stairs instead of the escalator or lift, or window-shop during your lunch hour. If you'd rather swim, cycle, do yoga, or dig in your garden, that's fine, too. Even standing at the ironing board while watching *EastEnders* on the television will burn calories. The point is, the more you move, the faster your sugar belly will melt away.

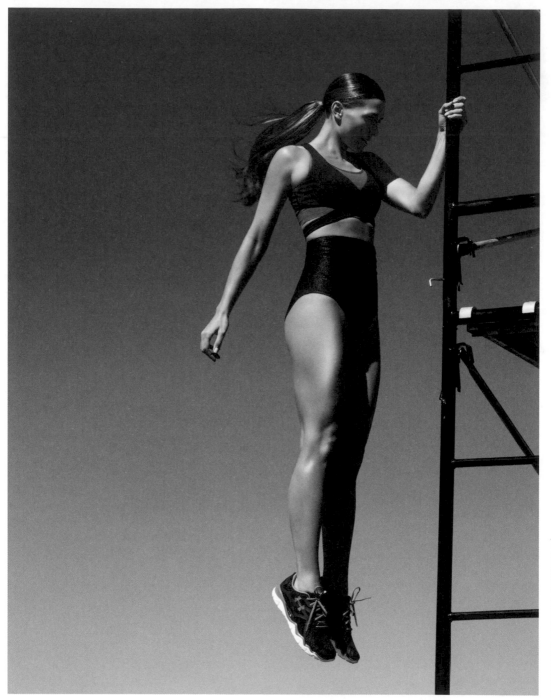

SUGAR-BELLY WORKOUTS

✦ FAST ROUTINES ✦ SOOTHING STRETCHES ✦

While the 20-day Shrink Your Sugar Belly plan will cut inches off your waistline, you can ramp up these results with this chapter. Mix and match these simple cardio, resistance and yoga routines to prime your mind and body to burn even more tummy fat and quieten your cravings. Get a move on, why don't you?

110 Fat-Burning Cardio
Get your heart pumping and speed up your metabolism by slotting these simple, do-anywhere exercises into your 20-day plan.

114 Tone-Up Resistance
How do you get your body burning belly fat, long after your workout has ended? Simple – work your muscles and they'll torch fat all day.

118 Energising Yoga
Slim down and get ready for the day with these high-pep stretches designed to boost your fat-burning and send sluggishness packing.

124 Relaxing Yoga
If cutting out your beloved sugar has you frazzled and fraught, try these stretches to soothe cravings and quieten a busy mind.

BURN
OFF YOUR
SUGAR
BELLY

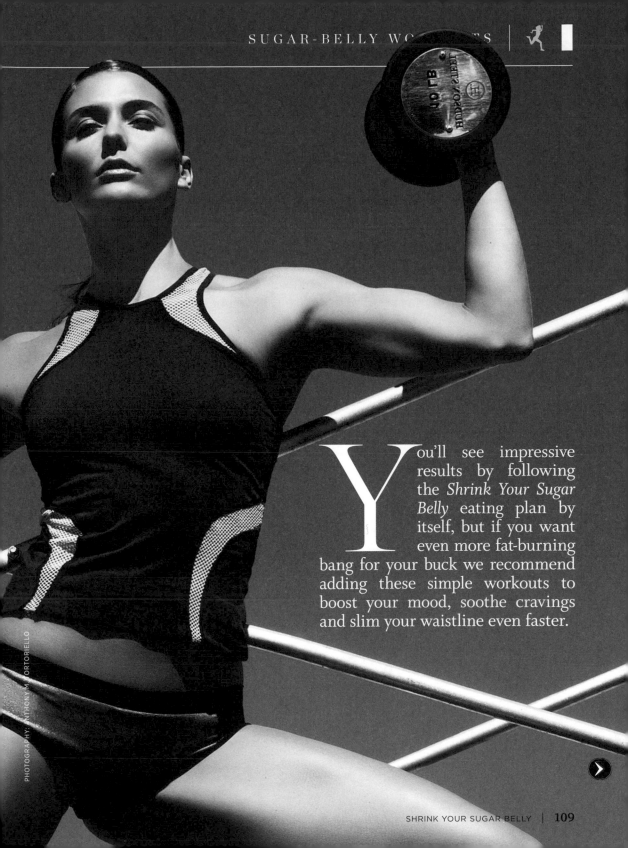

Y ou'll see impressive results by following the *Shrink Your Sugar Belly* eating plan by itself, but if you want even more fat-burning bang for your buck we recommend adding these simple workouts to boost your mood, soothe cravings and slim your waistline even faster.

THE TOTAL BODY TONER

Perform this routine at least twice a week. Do each exercise for the recommended number of reps, then repeat the set of exercises two more times. Use a weight that leaves you feeling fatigued at the end of each exercise – you can use a different amount of weight for different exercises, if needed. If you get tired on the second time, you may need to decrease the weight for your third go.

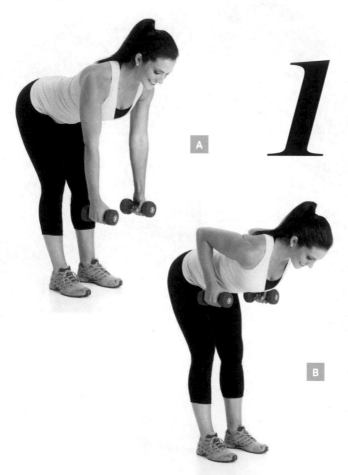

1 HINGE AND ROW

Stand with your feet about hip-width apart, holding the dumbbells with your arms at your sides. Keeping your abs tight and your chest lifted, bend at the hips and slowly lower until your torso is about parallel to the floor and the dumbbells hang beneath your shoulders **(A)**. Don't round your back. Bend your elbows and pull the dumbbells up towards your ribcage **(B)**. Lower the dumbbells and then stand back up. Do this 10 times.

CHEST PUMP

Lie on your back with your knees bent, feet flat on the floor. Hold the dumbbells by your shoulders, elbows pointing out to the sides **(A)**. Straighten your arms and press the dumbbells up over your chest **(B)**. When your arms are fully extended, lift your shoulders off the floor to press the dumbbells a little higher **(C)**. Hold for a second. Lower your shoulders, keeping your arms straight, then bend your arms to return to the start position. Do 10 times.

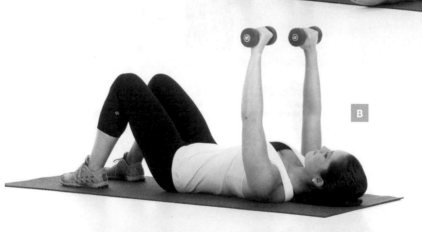

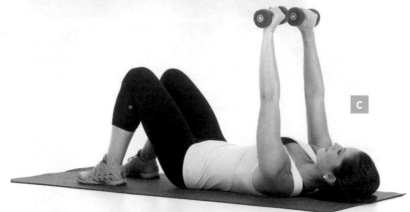

PHOTOGRAPHY: MITCH MANDELL

3

SIDE LUNGE WITH A CURL AND PRESS

Stand with your feet together and hold the dumbbells by your shoulders, arms bent and elbows pointing down **(A)**. Step your left foot out to the side and bend your left leg to sit back while keeping the right leg straight. As you lunge, extend your arms and lower the dumbbells **(B)**. Press into your left foot and straighten your leg to stand up. As you do that, bend your elbows and curl the dumbbells toward your shoulders, then press them overhead as you bring your feet back together **(C)**. Do 10 times, then repeat the lunge on the opposite side.

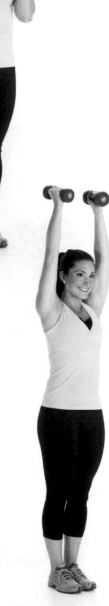

A

B

C

UPSWING

Stand with your feet about hip-width apart and hold a dumbbell down in front of you with both hands. Bend your hips and knees and sit back into a squat, lowering the dumbbell to the outside of your left leg **(A)**. As you stand up, raise the dumbbell diagonally across your body, keeping your arms extended, and rotate your torso to the right **(B)**. Do 10 times, then repeat, swinging your arms in the opposite direction.

4

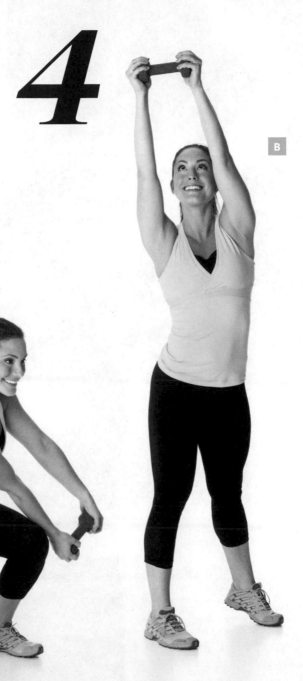

PHOTOGRAPHY: MITCH MANDELL

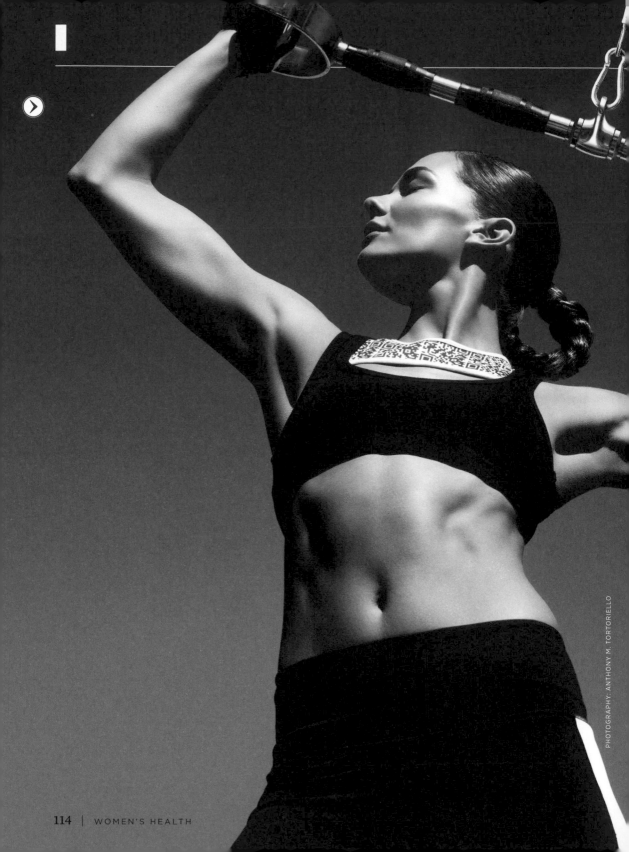

PHOTOGRAPHY: ANTHONY M. TORTORIELLO

THE SUGAR BELLY BLASTER

Do two sets of this series of exercises in order, with a 30-60 second rest and/or stretch between exercises. Do this routine at least twice a week

1 PELVIC TILTS

Lie face-up on the floor with your knees bent and feet flat on the floor **(A)**. Pull your navel towards your spine and curl your tailbone up towards the ceiling, lifting your hips slightly off the floor **(B)**. Hold for a second, then release **(C)**. Do 20 times.

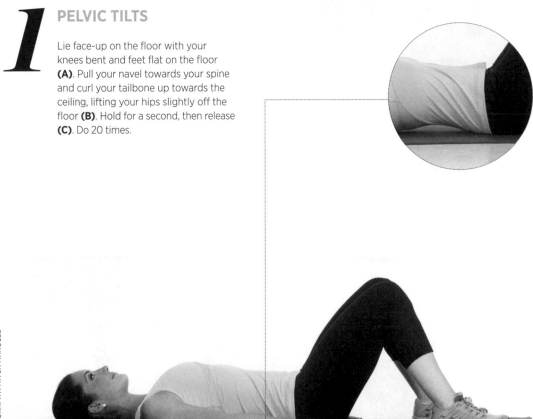

PHOTOGRAPHY: MITCH MANDELL

BICYCLE

Lie face up on the floor with your knees bent, feet flat on the floor, and hands behind your head. Raise your head and shoulders off the floor and twist to the right, bringing your right knee in towards your left elbow and extending your left leg at about a 45-degree angle. Lower and switch sides, twisting to the left and bringing your left knee and right elbow towards each other. Do 20 times, alternating sides. Each side counts as 1 rep.

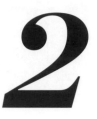

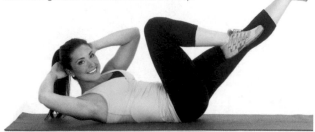

STANDING BALANCE

Balancing on one leg, swing your arms forward and back as vigorously as possible **(A)**. Next, alternate reaching one arm up overhead and lean to that side **(B)**. Then rotate your torso from side to side **(C)**. Do each of these moves 20 times, alternating arms. Each swing or twist counts as 1 rep. Switch legs and repeat. Finally, extend your arms overhead and diagonally to the left **(D)**, and pull your arms and right leg toward each other and then apart **(E)**. Do 10 times, then switch legs. Make it easier: take a break, putting your foot down in between moves. **Up the challenge** Stand on a pillow as you perform the moves.

3 SEATED BALANCE

Sit with your legs bent, feet on the floor, and grasp your hands behind your thighs. Shift your weight back onto your backside as you raise your feet so your calves are parallel to the floor. Once you've found your point of balance, extend your arms out in front of you. Keep your chest lifted and don't round your back. Hold for 1 minute. If needed, bring your legs down and take a break. Then hold again until your holding time adds up to 1 minute.

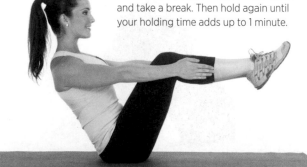

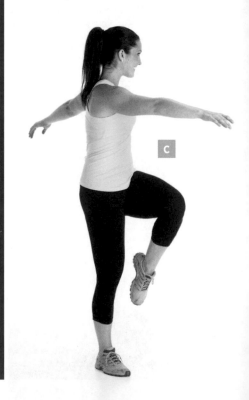

C

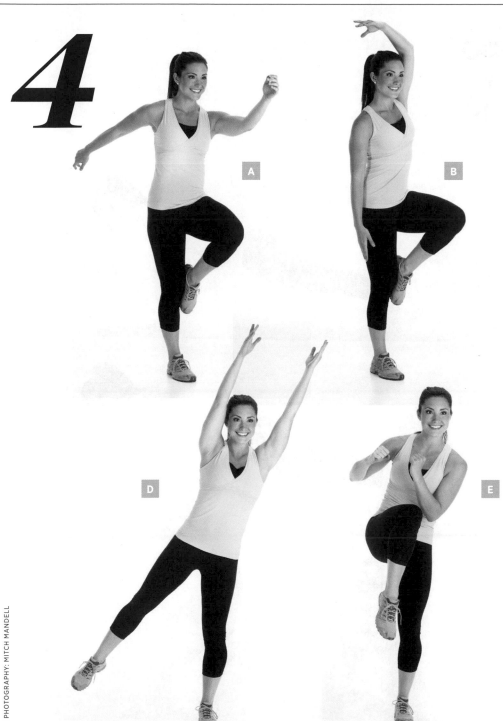

4

A

B

D

E

5

SHIFTING PLANK

Hold a push-up position, balancing on the balls of your feet and toes and your palms, hands directly beneath your shoulders **(A)**. Shift your weight forward **(B)**, to the left, and to the right **(C)**, without moving your hands. Hold each position for up to a count of 5 and return to centre in between each shift. Do 3 times. Make it easier: hold the plank without shifting. **Up the challenge** Raise one foot off the floor and then shift.

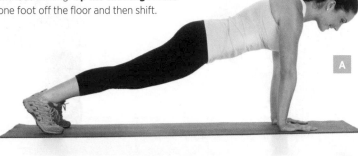

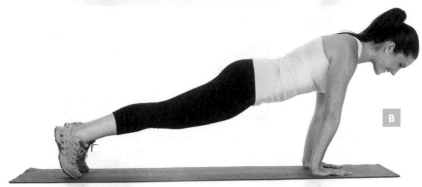

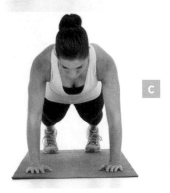
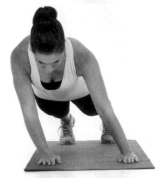

ENERGISING YOGA

Do two sets of this series of exercises in order. Rest and/or stretch for 30-60 seconds between exercises. Do this routine at least twice a week

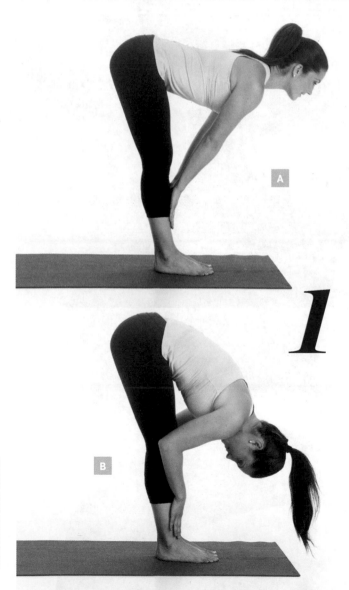

1

FORWARD BEND

Exhale and reach your arms out in front of you, palms down, as you bend forward from your hips, keeping your back flat and chest lifted as you lower until you're about parallel to the floor. Then curve your back and place your hands on your thighs, feet or floor – whatever is most comfortable **(A)**. Bend your knees slightly if you feel any strain. Inhale as you flatten your back and lift your head and chest up to look forward **(B)**. Exhale and curve your back to look at your legs. Inhale to stand up, circling your arms out to the sides and overhead, and then down to your sides. Repeat the Arm Circles and Forward Bend together 4 more times, but don't stand up on the final time through. Instead move into Plank.

PHOTOGRAPHY: MITCH MANDELL

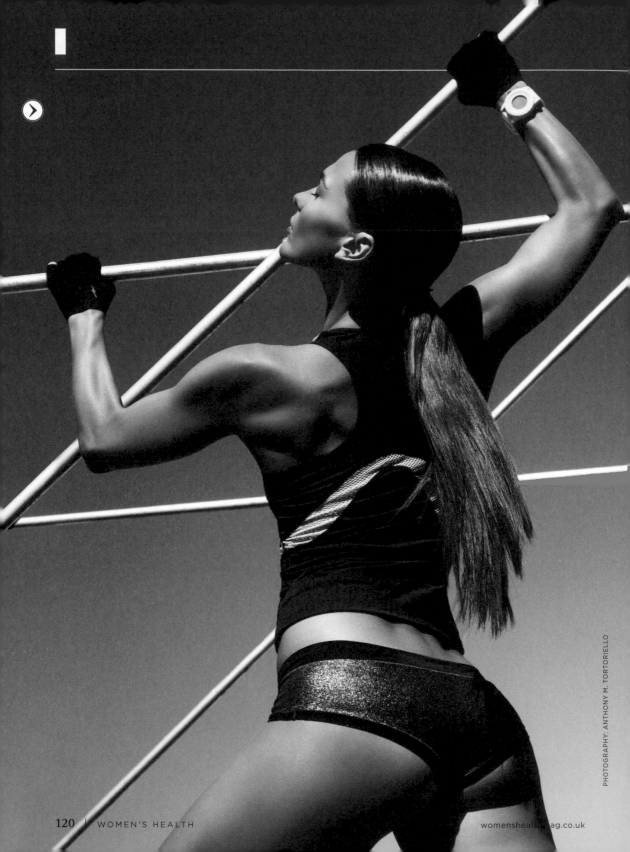

PHOTOGRAPHY: ANTHONY M. TORTORIELLO

2 MOUNTAIN

Stand tall with your feet together, toes forward and arms at your sides, palms in. Lift your chest and drop your shoulders back and down. Breathe deeply for 1 minute, pressing your feet into the floor and pushing the crown of your head towards the ceiling.

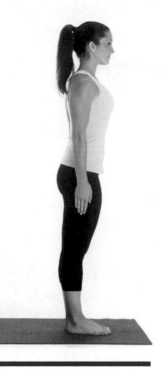

3 ARM CIRCLES

Inhale and raise your arms out to the sides, palms up, and circle them overhead. Exhale and lower them back to your sides. Repeat Arm Circles 4 more times, but don't lower your arms on the final time through. Instead, move into Forward Bend.

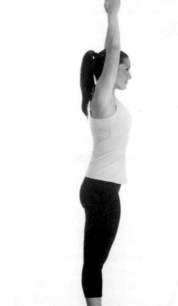

PHOTOGRAPHY: MITCH MANDELL

4 PLANK

Inhale and bend your knees and place your hands on the floor alongside your feet. Step your feet back one at a time and balance on your hands, your toes and the balls of your feet. Your hands should be directly beneath your shoulders. Your heels, ankles, bottom, spine, shoulders, neck and head should all be in line. Hold this position for 1 minute, if you can.

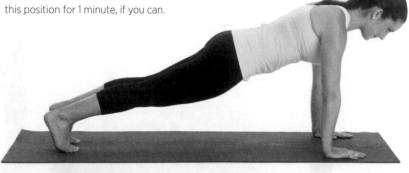

5 DOWNWARD-FACING DOG

As you exhale, move onto your toes and the balls of your feet. Lift your hips toward the ceiling and press back into an inverted V position. Hold for 5 breaths. On your next breath, walk your feet toward your hands, moving into a Forward Bend. Inhale and flatten your back, lifting your head and chest up as you look forward. Exhale and curve your back, looking at your legs. Inhale to stand up, circling your arms out to the sides and overhead, and then down to your sides into Mountain pose. Repeat the poses from Mountain through Downward-Facing Dog 4 more times (but without the repeats above). Remain in Downward-Facing Dog on the final time, then move into Crescent Lunge.

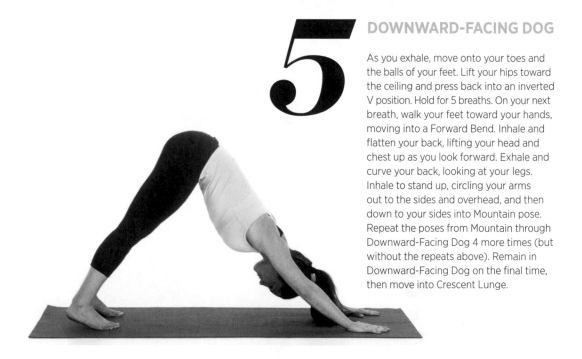

6

UPWARD-FACING DOG

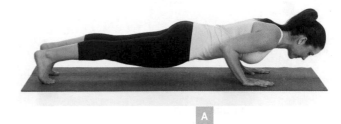

Exhale and bend your elbows back, keeping your arms close to your body, and slowly lower yourself to the floor, like you're doing a press-up **(A)**. With your toes pointed and palms on the floor in front of your shoulders, inhale and gently lift your upper body backoff the floor as far as comfortably possible, opening up your chest and pressing the tops of your feet into the floor **(B)**. Use your back muscles, not your hands, to lift.

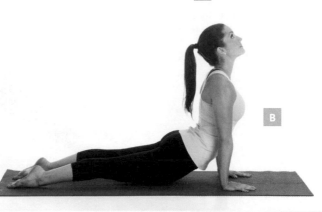

7

CRESCENT LUNGE

Inhale and lift your left leg behind you. As you exhale, swing it forward, stepping your left foot in between your hands. Inhale and bend your left knee, keeping it directly over your ankle, and raise your arms overhead. Make sure your toes point forward and your right heel is lifted off the floor.

PHOTOGRAPHY: MITCH MANDELL

8

WARRIOR 2

Exhale and lower your arms, turning your body toward the right, lowering your right heel, and angling your right toes toward the back right corner of the mat. Reach your arms out to the sides from your fingertips, looking toward your left hand.

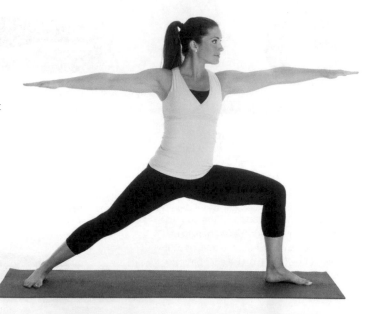

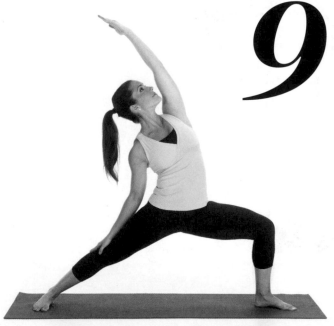

9

REVERSE WARRIOR

As you exhale, circle your right arm, placing your right hand on your right leg, and raise your left arm overhead, looking towards your left hand. Circle both hands down onto the floor on either side of your left foot. Step your left foot back into Plank pose. Repeat the poses from Plank (without the repeats) but lift your right leg when you are in Downward-Facing Dog in order to go into the Crescent Lunge pose on the opposite side. Then from Plank, do Upward- and Downward-Facing Dogs again, return to the Forward Bend, and finish in Mountain pose, breathing deeply for at least a minute.

RELAXING YOGA

Do two sets of this series of exercises in order. Rest and/or stretch for 30-60 seconds between exercises. Do this routine at least twice a week

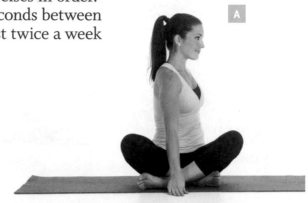

A

1

SEATED TWISTS & BENDS

Sit cross-legged with your hands out to your sides and your fingertips lightly touching the floor. Inhale and raise your arms overhead. As you exhale, twist to the left and lower your arms so the right one is in front of you (in the 12 o'clock position, if you were sitting on a clock) and the left one slightly behind you (in the 7 to 8 o'clock position) **(A)**. Repeat twisting to the opposite side. Do 20 in total, alternating sides. Face forward and recross your legs so the opposite one is in front. Reach your left arm up overhead and bend to the right as you inhale **(B)**, then return to start position as you exhale. Repeat on the opposite side. Do 20 in total, alternating sides. Walk your hands out in front of you and fold over your legs as far as is comfortable **(C)**. Hold for 8 deep breaths. Walk your hands back in and sit up. Then recross your legs and repeat.

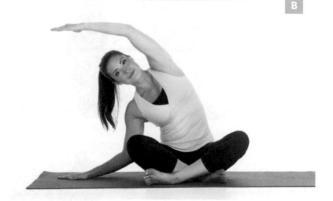

B

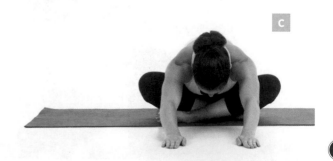

C

PHOTOGRAPHY: MITCH MANDELL

CAT COW STRETCHES

2

Shift forward so you're on all fours with your hands beneath your shoulders, your knees beneath your hips and your head in line with your spine. Inhale and lift your chest and tailbone towards the ceiling to arch your back **(A)**. Exhale and curve your back, tucking your tailbone and dropping your chin towards your chest **(B)**. As you inhale, sit back onto your heels, stretching your hips back and your arms forward **(C)**. Come back up to the start position as you exhale. Do 10 of these. Next, raise your right arm straight up to the ceiling, looking at your hand. Then sweep your arm down under your body and behind your left arm so your head and shoulder rest on the mat **(D)**. Hold for 3 to 5 breaths. Come back up and repeat with your left arm.

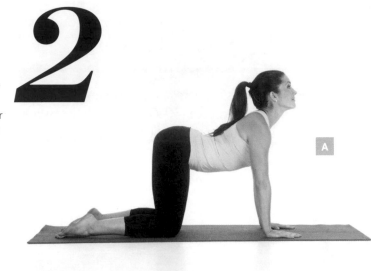

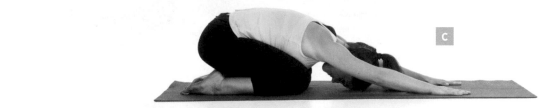

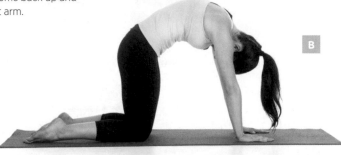

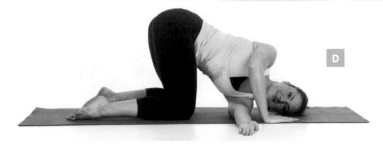

3 CORPSE POSE

Lie face-up on the floor with your arms extended and slightly angled away from your body, palms up. Your legs should be at a comfortable distance apart and relaxed so your feet roll out. Close your eyes and focus on your breathing for at least 3 minutes. You can put on some relaxing music or focus on a positive phrase such as "I am getting healthy" to enhance the effects. Feel free to stay in this pose for as long as you like.

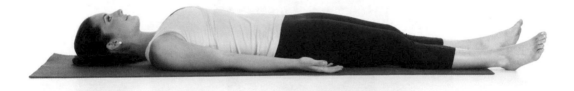

4 KNEE HUGS

Lie face-up on the floor and pull one leg into your chest, feeling the stretch in your back. You can lift your head off the floor and towards your knee for a deep stretch. Hold for 8 deep breaths. Release your leg and repeat with the opposite leg. Then pull both knees into your chest. Hold each position for 8 deep breaths.

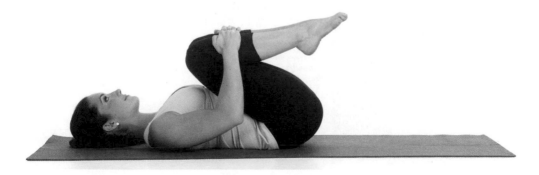

PHOTOGRAPHY: MITCH MANDELL

Perfect
10

POWER SHAKES

*For some of us, a shiny new gym membership is for January.
But a solid, 60-second protein-shake recipe? Well, that's for life*

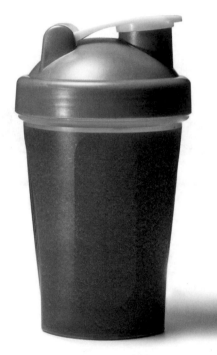

PSYCLE'S SMOOTH RED VELVET SHAKE

Serves 1 | 380 cals
0.3g sat fat | 30.8g protein

INGREDIENTS

❋ 1 scoop of **Chocolate Vega
Sport Performance Protein**
❋ 1 cooked **beetroot** ❋ ½ cup
raspberries ❋ ½ frozen **banana**
❋ Handful **spinach** ❋ 200ml
unsweetened almond milk

METHOD

London's coolest spinning-meets-meditation
studio does one of the best shakes we've
ever tasted. Almost better than a real red
velvet cake. You know the drill: chop and
blend everything. **Smoothie operator:**
Beetroot is loaded with antioxidants and
ups nitric oxide, which enhances oxygen
transportation to muscles to increase
endurance pre-exercise. Beet that.

PHOTOGRAPHY: ANTHONY SERGIEW

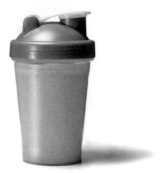

BODYISM'S WAKEY-WAKEY MORNING-BOOST SHAKE

Serves 1 | 507 cals | 5.3g sat fat | 21.4g protein

✳ 1 **green teabag** ✳ 3 tbsps **hot water** ✳ 1 tsp **honey** ✳ 200ml **water**, **almond milk** or **rice milk** ✳ 1 scoop **Bodyism Body Brilliance Powder** ✳ 3 **brazil nuts** ✳ Handful **sunflower seeds** ✳ Handful **pumpkin seeds**

Bodyism, run by *WH* contributor James Duigan, is the gym of supermodels. To get a taste of Rosie Huntington-Whiteley's favourite, brew the teabag, remove it and stir in the honey before blending it with all the other ingredients until smooth. Beautiful. **Smoothie operator:** The nuts' anti-inflammatory omega-3s mean this is like a facial in a glass.

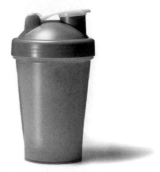

GRACE BELGRAVIA'S BERRY YOU-MAKE-ME-BLUSH SHAKE

Serves 1 | 851 cals | 13.8g sat fat | 37.1g protein

✳ 50g fresh mixed **berries** ✳ 1 **banana** ✳ ½ cup **porridge oats** ✳ 1 tbsp **hemp protein powder** ✳ 400ml **almond milk** ✳ 3 tbsps **Greek yoghurt** ✳ 1 tbsp **flaxseed** ✳ 1 tbsp **Jax Coco coconut oil**

This glitzy private-members' club-come-gym is the place to 'sweatwork' (that's network while you workout, FYI). The calorie count in this decadent shake makes it a meal in one. Just blend and pour. Done! **Smoothie operator:** Flaxseed is the star player in this shake; it has more protein than eggs. Find it a bit hard to digest? Go for chia seeds instead.

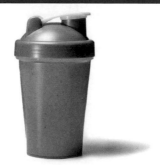

FRAME'S TOTALLY LEAN, MEAN, GREEN MACHINE SHAKE

Serves 1 | 328 cals | 1.4g sat fat | 19.1g protein

✳ 50g **watercress** ✳ ¼ **avocado** ✳ ½ **apple** ✳ 1 tsp **turmeric** ✳ 1 inch **ginger** ✳ ½ **banana** ✳ 30g **hemp protein** ✳ 250ml **coconut water**

If you're a hipster who's into fitness, you'll love Frame in east London. And you'll be frothing over this green shake – it's that good. But if you can't hotfoot it to Frame, simply combine all these ingredients together and blend until smooth. If you need to, add more coconut water and re-blend. **Smoothie operator:** With its mix of proteins, fats and complex carbohydrates, it's a completely balanced meal – ideal if you tend to opt for a light lunch.

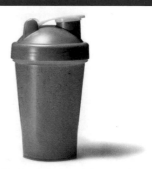

LOMAX'S FIVE-A-DAY-FOR-WORK-AND-PLAY BOOSTER SHAKE

Serves 1 | 198 cals | 0.3g sat fat | 4.1g protein

✳ 1 scoop **Warrior NRG protein powder** ✳ Juice 1 **beetroot** ✳ 2 **apples** ✳ 1 **carrot** ✳ 1 inch **ginger** ✳ 1 **lemon** ✳ Handful **spinach**

This Chelsea super gym is behind some of London's most envied bodies. It also knows how to make a very mean protein shake. Add the powder to the beetroot juice, pop in a blender and blitz the rest of the ingredients and blitz away! And you're halfway to gorgeous. **Smoothie operator:** This is the perfect pre-training meal. Full of starchy vegetables to charge your workout, vegan protein powder is highly digestible so you can easily absorb its nutrients.

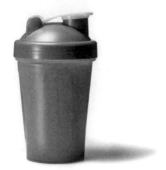

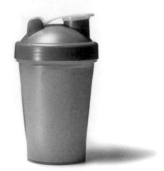

EQUINOX'S ULTIMATE ENERGY GO BANANAS AND BLUEBERRY SHAKE

Serves 1 | 282 cals | 0g sat fat | 32.1g protein

✳ 1 **banana** ✳ Handful **blueberries** ✳ 1 scoop **vanilla protein** ✳ 160ml **coconut water** ✳ 1 tsp **maca** ✳ 4 **ice cubes**

This US luxury gym chain has been churning out body beautifuls for years. Its secret? This shake. Put the ice in first so it hits the blades quicker, then put everything else on top and blend for 1 minute. Easy. **Smoothie operator:** Post-gym, the coconut water rehydrates while maca strengthens bones and muscles. Down in one.

BARRY'S BOOTCAMP PEANUT BUTTER SHAKE

Serves 1 | 372 cals | 1.7g sat fat | 36.5g protein

✳ 230ml **almond milk** ✳ Handful frozen **strawberries** ✳ Handful frozen **blueberries** ✳ 1 tbsp **Meridian peanut butter** ✳ 1 scoop **vanilla protein** ✳ Several **ice cubes**

There's a reason why the Beckhams are fans of this hard-core club – probably something to do with this shake. It's as sweet and delicious as David. **Smoothie operator:** Because peanuts aren't actually nuts, but legumes (the same family as lentils and chickpeas), they're packed with protein – around 7g per tablespoon.

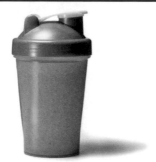

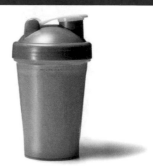

THE MOVEMENT'S GO COCO ON PINA COLADA POWER SHAKE

Serves 1 | 152 cals | 0.2g sat fat | 19g protein

✳ 1 frozen **banana** ✳ 300ml **coconut water** ✳ Splash **pineapple juice** ✳ Handful **ice** ✳ 1 scoop **pea protein powder**

Straight from one of the most exclusive gyms in New York, this smoothie is full of electrolytes to help you refuel and prevent muscle cramps during exercise. We'll take two, please. **Smoothie operator:** Pineapple is full of bromelain, an enzyme that helps digestion. It's particularly concentrated in the pineapple stalk, so if you're juicing from fresh, chuck that in, too. Sounds weird, but trust us on this one.

CHHP'S IT-WAS-MINT-TO-BE CHOCOLATE CASHEW SHAKE

Serves 1 | 290 cals | 1.5g sat fat | 28.3g protein

✳ 25g **chocolate whey protein powder** ✳ 15g **cashews** ✳ 200ml **hazelnut milk** ✳ 3g **mint leaves**

The Centre For Health and Human Performance (CHHP) takes training to the next level. And this protein shake is one of its secret weapons. You know what to do... blend it in one! For a smoother texture, strain ingredients through a sieve. **Smoothie operator:** If you like your workouts tough, then this drink is for you. Hazelnuts are full of copper and manganese, both exercise essentials because they help iron absorption for energy and bone formation for strength.

DAVID BARTON'S PUMP IT UP

Serves 1 | 291 cals
1g sat fat | 29g protein

INGREDIENTS

✳ 4 **ice cubes** ✳ $^3/4$ cup **water** ✳ 1 scoop **Cellucor Cinnamon Swirl whey protein** powder ✳ $^1/2$ tsp **ginger powder** ✳ 1/4 tsp **cinnamon** ✳ 1 tbsp **molasses** ✳ 4 large slices **cooked** pumpkin, pureed ✳ $^1/2$ tsp **vanilla extract**

METHOD

David Barton Gyms in the US are possibly the hippest spaces ever. Not surprising when they're serving shakes like this. **Smoothie operator:** Rich in A and B vitamins, pumpkin is the perfect post-exercise food – combined with the protein powder you use, it's ideal for muscle repair.

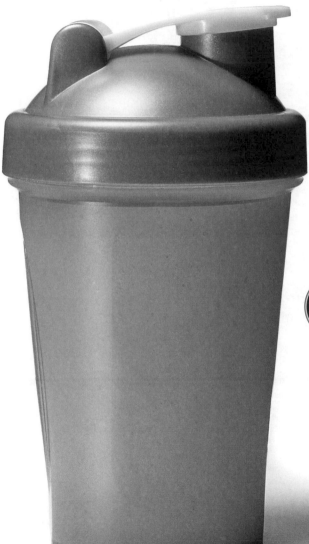

Tricks to Try

AMINO GIRLS LOOK YOUNGER

Want to slow down ageing? Look no further than your daily shake

Scientists at the University of Milan found that consuming amino acids can lengthen your lifespan by up to 12%. The magical protein building blocks digested when you drink one shake a day increase activation of your cells' mitochondria, which in turn slow the ageing process. Count us in.

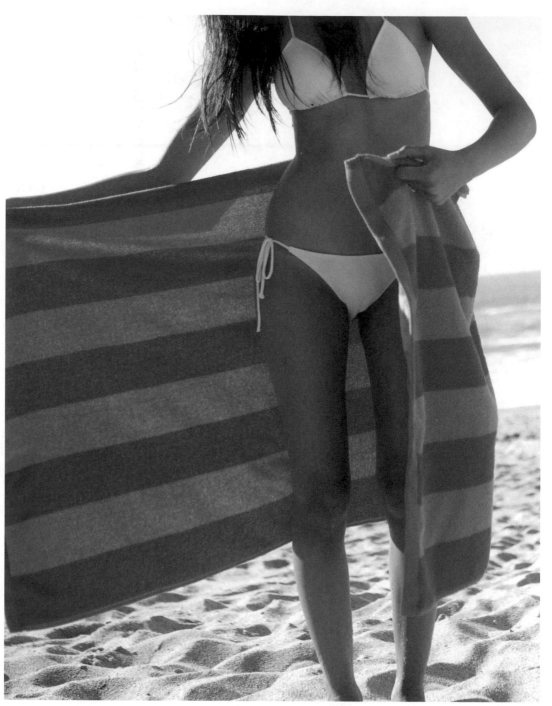

6

LOW SUGAR
FOR LIFE

+ EXERCISE CHOICE + RE-INTRODUCE + ENJOY! +

Now you've reset your formerly overloaded taste buds and started shedding your sugar belly, it's entirely possible to let sweets back into your life. But how can you enjoy sugar without the addiction kicking in again? Follow our smart strategies for a careful re-introduction and kick self-denial into touch – then savour every mouthful.

134 Hello, Sugar!
If you choose to let the sweet stuff back into your diet, you're going to have to do it carefully – and cleverly. Here's how to enjoy treats without slipping back into old habits.

138 Live the Sweet Life For Good
Keep losing weight, bring skin back to its best and harness all that extra energy: here's all the expert tips and motivation you'll need to continue enjoying life the sugar-smart way.

142 Suss Out Hidden Sugars
It's easy enough to control the obviously sugary treats in your diet – it's the sneaky ones you have to watch out for! Wise up, become a label queen and keep your sugar belly away.

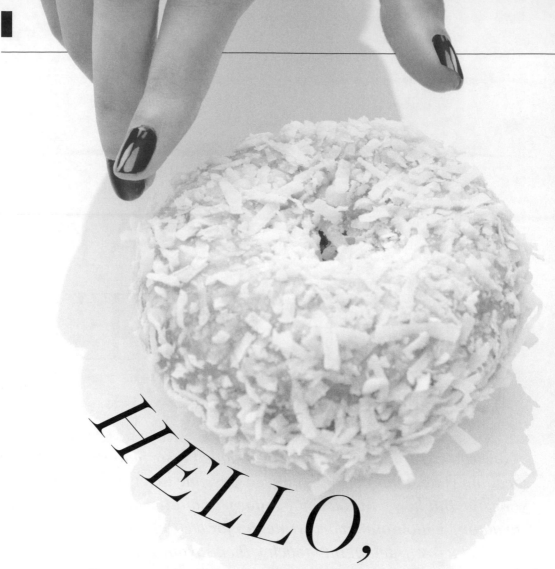

HELLO,

By now, you should have a noticeably slimmer middle and a new outlook

ou've come a long way, baby! You've fended off cravings, maybe even battled tiredness and mood swings, and all to kick your sugar habit. Now for the enjoyable, delicious part, where you reintroduce sugar simply for the pleasure of having it. At the beginning of this book, we told you that we didn't want to banish it from your life forever; a little added sugar in your diet every day (if you still want it!) is perfectly fine. We define 'a little' as no more than six teaspoons a day (24 grams) of added sugar.

PHOTOGRAPHY: GETTY IMAGES

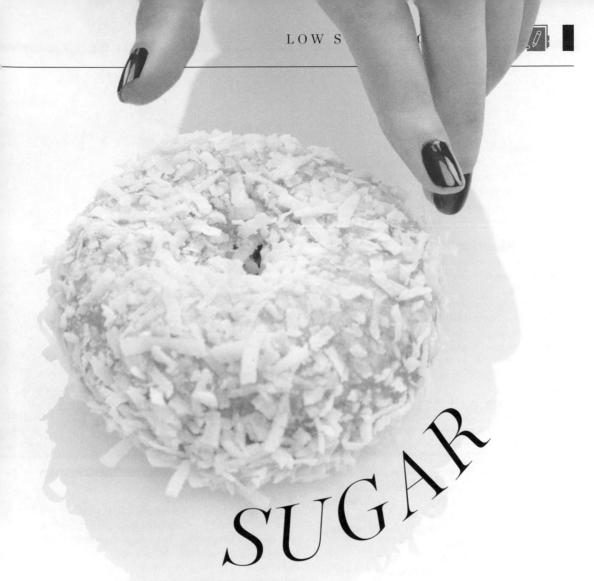

SUGAR

on sugar. Are you ready to let it safely back into your life? We show you how

This doesn't include the sugar that's in whole foods naturally – we're talking about the stuff that gets added to processed foods and beverages and what you sprinkle, mix and stir yourself. Look at it this way: two small chocolate-chip cookies have seven grams of sugar, less in total than the nine grams found naturally in a medium orange – but all of the sugar in the cookies is added, so makes up some of your day's 24-gram allowance. The orange is fine.

Until now, you've been eating under six teaspoons of added sugar a day, so you know that a sugar belly-

shrinking way of eating can be tasty and satisfying. But you might like to have a sweet treat here or there. The good news is that you can and still stay within the six-teaspoon daily limit.

For instance, maybe you'll choose to add a teaspoon of sugar (four grams) to your coffee and drizzle a teaspoon of maple syrup (four more) on your oatmeal in the morning; have a hamburger on a bun (three grams) with a tablespoon of ketchup (four grams) at lunch; and half a bag of Maltesers as your sweet treat (10 grams), for a total of 25 grams or just a smidgen over six teaspoons of sugar. That's perfectly OK. Staying slim, healthy, energetic and sugar smart for life means being aware of where the sugar lurks in your diet and making informed choices.

Reconsidering sugar

At this point, you're hopefully noticing a lot of changes: energy, up. Mood, brighter. Skin, clearer. Sugar cravings, crushed. You're now experiencing the benefits of nutritional balance – more whole foods and fresh flavours, and significantly less sugar and refined starches. And, more to the point, the pounds around your waist should be melting away, too.

Now that those zero-sugar days are conquered and you can bring sugar back into your diet, you probably feel one of three ways: not really missing it (perhaps to your surprise), excited to be able to have treats again, or wondering whether you'll be able to reintroduce treats without sliding back into old eating patterns. Sugary foods have not been a part of your diet now for two weeks, so you're in a perfect position to decide what part they'll play in your future.

To do so, remember all the sugar sources you identified as 'must have' on the first day of the Sugar Step-Down. How often do you think about them? Then have a small portion of one of them as you work through the following stages:

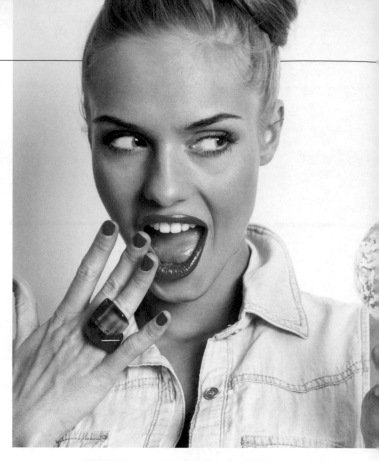

1 Look at your treat

Note your level of anticipation. Recall what you liked about it and how it used to make you feel when you ate it (positive or negative). Compare those feelings to the way you've been feeling since it's been out of your diet. How do you think having the treat will change that? Are you looking forward to your first bite? What do you expect to feel after you eat it?

2 Take a bite

Nice and slowly. Notice the flavour and the texture. Does it taste the way you remembered it? Are you getting a rush of pleasure?

3 Eat the rest of your treat slowly

Continue to focus on flavour and texture. Do you like what you're eating? Did you miss it? Would you still say that this is one of your favourite treats?

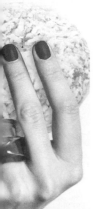

Try this exercise with a few different sugar sources during this week and see how your reactions vary. There aren't any right or wrong answers – the point is to make you aware of the effect sugar has on you. Before you started the *Shrink Your Sugar Belly* plan, treating yourself with Straight-Up Sugars or Sugar Mimics may have been part of your everyday habits. But now you've broken the habit, found other ways to cope with stress and stabilised your metabolism.

If your key sugar sources are still as satisfying as remembered, then have them in a reasonable way. If you can limit yourself to a small portion of 100-150 calories, then you can have one of them every day.

If you instead find that your must-have sugar sources no longer bring you much pleasure, but you'd still like to have some treats in your life, then experiment with some of the delicious dessert options in Chapter 8.

If you find that your favourite sugar sources trigger cravings, hunger or other symptoms, consider replacing them with other sweets and continue the process of carefully monitoring your mind and body's responses. And if you discover that sugar overall has lost its allure – just don't have it. Read on for some tasty, healthy recipes and get on with the Sweet Life!

4 After you're finished

Take a few minutes to consider whether you feel the way you thought you would when you started eating. Did the treat live up to your expectations? Do you want more right away or are you happy with the amount you had? Would you have been just as satisfied with something else?

5 Over the next hour

Watch your reactions to it carefully. Are you hungry sooner than you might have been otherwise? Do you feel cravings for that treat or another sugary food? Are you feeling headachey or a little tired? Or do you feel good physically and pleased that you've treated yourself to something you love?

Tricks to Try

GO TO THE DARK SIDE   It's the chocolate that's safe to indulge in

Good for the heart, good for the soul, maybe even good for your sugar belly! Dark chocolate is a great better-for-you treat. Swap it for milk chocolate and you'll consume significantly less sugar. But that's not the only reason we swoon for it. Although its flavour isn't traditionally sweet, its health benefits are.

Compared to milk chocolate, dark chocolate promotes that 'I'm-full' feeling known as satiety, lowers the desire to eat sweets and reduces calorie intake, which may help with weight loss, a study published in *Nutrition & Diabetes* found. When researchers gave participants 100g of either dark or milk chocolate and offered them pizza two hours later, those who consumed the dark chocolate ate 15 per cent fewer calories from the pizza than those who had milk chocolate.

If you're used to milk chocolate, go dark gradually to train your taste buds to appreciate the stronger taste. Pick a variety that has a 70 per cent or higher cocoa content and lists it as its first ingredient.

LIVE THE

SWEET LIFE
FOR GOOD

This newly slim waistline and dewy skin are yours for keeps if you stick to our six rules for sugar-smart living. Enjoy every mouthful and feel fantastic – for life

Y ou've got strategies to crush cravings. Coping techniques to cool your emotional connection with sugar. Tips to sleep better, relax more, move daily and enjoy life. As you prepare to strike out on your own, team the strategies you've been using throughout the plan with these big-picture strategies. Together, they'll help you stick to – and love – your sweet, sugar-smart life!

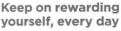
1 Keep on rewarding yourself, every day

By now, using your personal Reward Card has hopefully become a habit, and one that's had a real impact on your life. Don't give up doing that just because we've come to the end of the eating plan. In addition to helping you make your overall wellbeing a priority, treating yourself in non-food-based ways can benefit every area of your life.

2 Make breakfast a must

And here we go, banging on about breakfast again. But that's because it's so important! Metabolism revver. Brain booster. Cravings crusher; breakfast is all of those things. So whether you've lost the weight you want or are still working on it, continue to eat breakfast each day, and make sure it contains 15 to 20 grams of lean protein. Feel free to enjoy your favourite breakfasts from any part of this book, and stock your fridge, freezer and cupboards with cravings-crushing breakfast ingredients like sugar-free peanut butter, eggs and frozen edamame.

3 Forget about your sugar grams – just once a week

It's your birthday or someone else's, and there's cake. You're visiting the town with the best ice-cream place on the planet. You're at a restaurant where the desserts are to die for. Or maybe you just want a nice cold glass of lemonade on a hot day.

We don't expect you to fret about parcelling out a portion of that sugary treat that has exactly 150 calories and 12 grams of added sugar. Just have it – as long as you splurge only once a week and skip your daily 150-calorie indulgence that day.

The first few times, carefully monitor how you feel afterwards – physically and emotionally. Sometimes, you'll experience intense sugar cravings the day after you've had an anything-goes meal. Plan ahead, indulge, enjoy – and then clear your system of that sugar load by sticking to some Phase 1 or 2 recipes that day, and perhaps even the next.

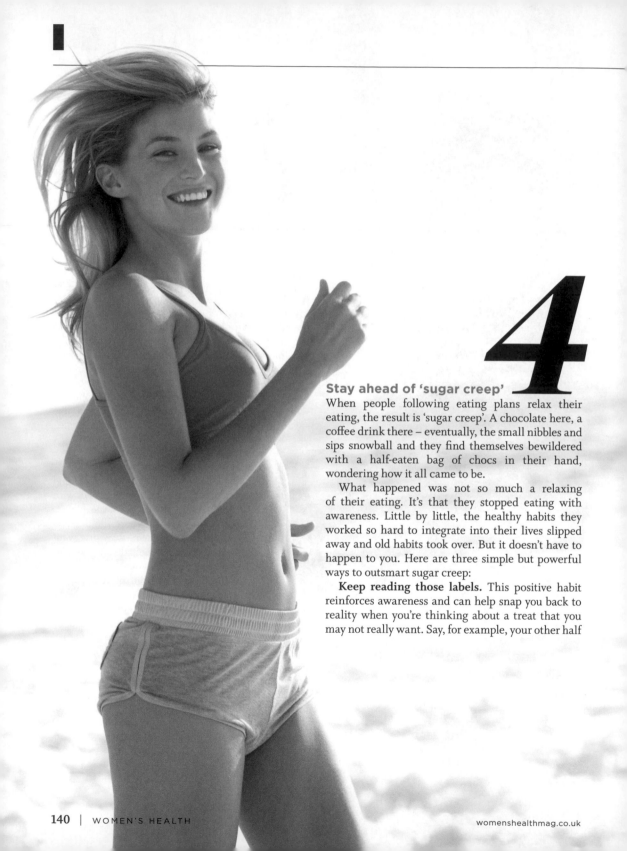

4

Stay ahead of 'sugar creep'

When people following eating plans relax their eating, the result is 'sugar creep'. A chocolate here, a coffee drink there – eventually, the small nibbles and sips snowball and they find themselves bewildered with a half-eaten bag of chocs in their hand, wondering how it all came to be.

What happened was not so much a relaxing of their eating. It's that they stopped eating with awareness. Little by little, the healthy habits they worked so hard to integrate into their lives slipped away and old habits took over. But it doesn't have to happen to you. Here are three simple but powerful ways to outsmart sugar creep:

Keep reading those labels. This positive habit reinforces awareness and can help snap you back to reality when you're thinking about a treat that you may not really want. Say, for example, your other half brings home a raspberry and cream-cheese Danish pastry. The label says that one serving has 15 grams of sugar. That's just short of four teaspoons – most of your daily allowance! Do you really, really, really want that pastry or would a few squares of dark chocolate or a slice of wholegrain toast with 100 per cent raspberry spread hit the spot just as well?

Plan your treats. For the most part, you should decide what you'll have as a treat on any particular day and stick to that. The idea is to limit your spontaneous sugar indulgences as much as possible. Planning not only helps you manage your intake of sugar but increases your enjoyment of it when you decide to indulge.

When you treat yourself, do it mindfully. Every day, give your full attention to the first bite of the sugary treat you've chosen for the day. Gaze at it lovingly. Sigh over it. Give thanks for it and give thought to its colour, scent, temperature and complexity of flavours. It's a way to pay respect to sugar and keep your awareness of its presence in your diet sharp. Sugar creep won't be able to gain the upper hand.

5. Have a plan for backsliding

What if, despite your best intentions, sugar does creep up on you? If you're staying aware of your sugar intake, you can nip it in the bud using this book. Simply go back to Phase 1 for a week or two to reset your sugar taste buds, then either progress through Phase 2 in the same way you did before – or just carry on with our healthy recipes from Chapter 6 onwards.

Planning doesn't only help you manage your intake of sugar, but increases your enjoyment when you decide to indulge

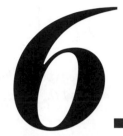

6. Savour life as much as you do sugar

We've been talking about savouring sweet foods – and now they're occasional treats you certainly will! But there are other things to savour. Take a moment to think about your schedule. Does it include activities that put a curl in your toes, get you really stoked and, overall, just glad to be alive?

This isn't ho-hum downtime in front of the telly enjoyment – we're talking real, unashamed pleasure. The more you indulge in pleasure in healthy ways, the less you'll look for it in sugar.

And the more laughter and joy you can add to your life, the less you'll feel you need to look for from food. But there is another, lesser-known dimension to pleasure: savouring. And research suggests it might be the key to true happiness.

In a study published in the *Journal of Positive Psychology*, researchers had participants keep diaries for 30 days. They recorded 'pleasant events' and how much they savoured them. Savourers got more pleasure by stopping to focus on a good thing, telling someone else about it or even screaming in delight. Wet-blanket types killed the joy by complaining that it could have been better, they didn't deserve it or it was almost over. But ultimately, savourers got the biggest happiness boost from pleasurable moments.

The skill set for good savouring is one part wild abandon (think of how an animal would eat something really, really tasty) and one part mature wisdom (using your mindful eating skills). Whether you're one or the other, practising the fine art of savouring can help you keep sugar in its rightful place in your life. Enjoy, enjoy and enjoy again.

SUSS OUT
ADDED SUGARS

Your Sweet Life secret weapon? That'll be the label. Learn how to decode packaging and you'll spot the sugar before it sneaks onto your midriff

Now that you're free to enjoy up to six teaspoons of added sugars (24 grams) a day (or, incidentally, an unfair nine teaspoons for men) in any way your heart desires, you'll need to keep track of how much you're eating.

Sometimes, 'sugar maths' is easy. Stir a teaspoon of the sweet stuff into your coffee or drizzle a teaspoon of honey on your morning porridge and you've consumed four grams of sugar, or one-sixth of your daily allowance.

But as we've mentioned before, determining the amount of added sugars in packaged or prepared foods can be tricky. Food manufacturers aren't required to separate naturally occurring and added sugars on their labels. What they list is the product's total sugars, which can come from the sugars naturally in the food, added sugars, or both.

Sneaky! But not sneaky enough. Here's a quick-and-dirty way to estimate any food's added sugars. On the product's Nutrition Facts label, look for Total Sugars.

If the product contains sugar, consider all of it to be added unless the food contains a significant amount of fruit, milk or yoghurt, or 'sweeter' vegetables such as carrots, corn, peas, sweet potatoes and winter squash.

MUST-READS Here's what to look for on the side of the packet

A	B	C
'of which sugars'	**Ingredients**	
If the label says it contains 0 grams of sugar (or a minimal amount, say up to three grams) – you're in the clear. Anything more and you'll need to look at the ingredients list.	Look at the product's ingredients list. Do you spot any form of added sugar? No? Then the sugar is naturally present in the food. Two examples: plain yoghurt or unsweetened apple sauce.	If you spot sugar or its aliases, it's time for some detective work. Once you're familiar with how much natural sugar unsweetened foods contain, it's simple to guesstimate how much added sugar the sweetened versions have.

NUTRITION

TYPICAL VALUES

	100g contains	Each biscuit contains	%GDA*	GDA* for a typical adult
Energy	2080kJ	240kJ		
	500kcal	60kcal	3%	2,000kcal
Protein	5.1g	0.6g		
Carbohydrates	67.9g	7.9g		
of which sugars	28.4g	3g Ⓐ	6%	50g
Fat	23g	3g	4%	70g
of which saturates	13.7g	2g	10%	20g
mono-unsaturates	6.7g	0.8g		
polyunsaturates	2g	0.2g		
Fibre	2.1g	0.2g		
Sodium	0.2g	trace		
Salt equivalent	0.5g	trace	<1%	6g

*Guideline daily amounts

INGREDIENTS

Ⓑ

Ⓒ Wheat flour, sugar, vegetable oil, whey solids, glucose syrup, wheat starch, salt, raising agents (ammonium bicarbonate, sodium bicarbonate), corn starch, vanillin, natural flavouring

**CONTAINS: WHEAT, MILK, GLUTEN
MAY ALSO CONTAIN TRACES OF NUTS**

500g

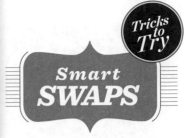

Tricks to Try

Smart SWAPS

Us Brits consume about 34 teaspoons of sugar a day. Roll back your intake with these tips from Mike Roussell, author of *The Six Pillars of Nutrition*

KICK THE CAN OF POP
Save 10 tsps

First swap it with diet pop to cut calories while still having your sweetness fix. Then, after a week or so, make the switch to fizzy water with a slice of lemon or lime.

SWEETEN YOGHURT NATURALLY
Save 2-4 tsps

Fruit-on-the-side yoghurts can contain almost 30g of sugar, much of it added. Opt for plain yoghurts and mix in blueberries or other fruit – or sprinkle on cinnamon for some fat-burning flavour.

SNACK ON WHOLE FOODS AND WHOLEGRAINS
Save 2-10 tsps

Instead of energy bars, sweets and biscuits, eat nuts, vegetables, and fibre-rich fruits (like apples, pears and berries) or wholegrains, like air-popped popcorn.

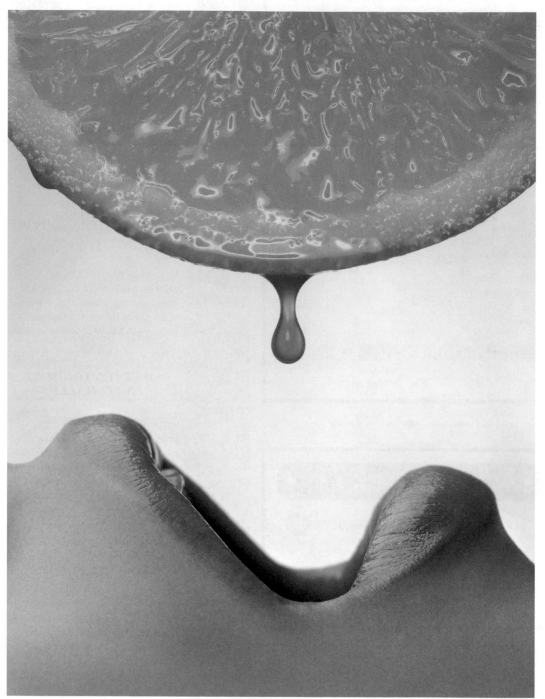

SWEET LIFE
MORNINGS

✦ BREAKFASTS ✦ BRUNCHES ✦ SMOOTHIES ✦

Get your first meal right and you'll stand a better chance of staying on track through the rest of the day. There are sugar-belly breakfast traps everywhere, from tempting pastries to deceptive shop-bought fruit smoothies – but this chapter has the recipes you need to stop unwanted sugar putting the dampeners on a really spectacular day

146 Breakfast fillers
Get the best possible start to your day – minimise added sugar content with these healthy versions of popular breakfast staples.

154 Super smoothies
Ditch the hidden calories of post-gym and café blends! Keep the health benefits *and* save money when you BIY (that's Blend It Yourself).

158 Power juices
Blending, not juicing, keeps the fibre you need to balance sugar spikes. Discover the dream combination for every mind, body and beauty goal.

162 It's shot o'clock!
Small is beautiful with the newest juice trend – learn how to nab the nutrients while ditching the usual fast-burn fruit sugar content.

CRAVINGS CHA

LEADING-LADY CROQUE MADAME

SERVES **2** · CALS **486** · SAT FAT **7.5g** · READY IN **30**MIN

WHY

When it comes to grab-and-go meals, you can't beat a sarnie. Wholewheat sourdough bread will keep you from feeling bloated, but its fibre combined with egg protein will fill you till lunch. The calcium in gruyere is great for your bones, nails and hair while cayenne boosts the flavour – and your body's fat-burning abilities, according to the *Journal of Proteome Research*.

INGREDIENTS

- 2 tsps **olive oil**
- 1 small **onion**
- Juice of 2 **lemons**
- 2 tsps **olive oil**
- ½ bunch **kale**
- Pinch of **cayenne**
- Pinch of **nutmeg**
- 4 thin slices **wholewheat sourdough bread**
- 60g **gruyere**
- 60g lean, deli-sliced **ham**
- 2 **eggs**

METHOD

1/ Cook the onion for 8 minutes. Add the kale, cayenne, nutmeg and 3 tbsps of water. Cook until the kale is tender – around 7 to 8 minutes. Season with salt and pepper.
2/ Sprinkle two slices of bread with about 15g of the cheese. Then top each slice with half of the ham, half of the kale-onion mix and another 15g of the cheese. Place the remaining slices on top. Almost there.
3/ Cook the sandwiches in a lightly greased, non-stick frying pan until golden brown.
4/ Remove the sandwiches. Fry two eggs and place one on top of each sandwich to serve.

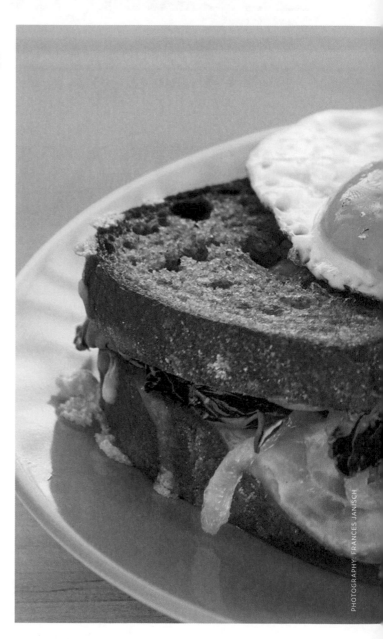

PHOTOGRAPHY: FRANCES JANISCH

SERS

A good breakfast is your first defence against temptation. Load up on protein or choose low-sugar alternatives to sweet favourites

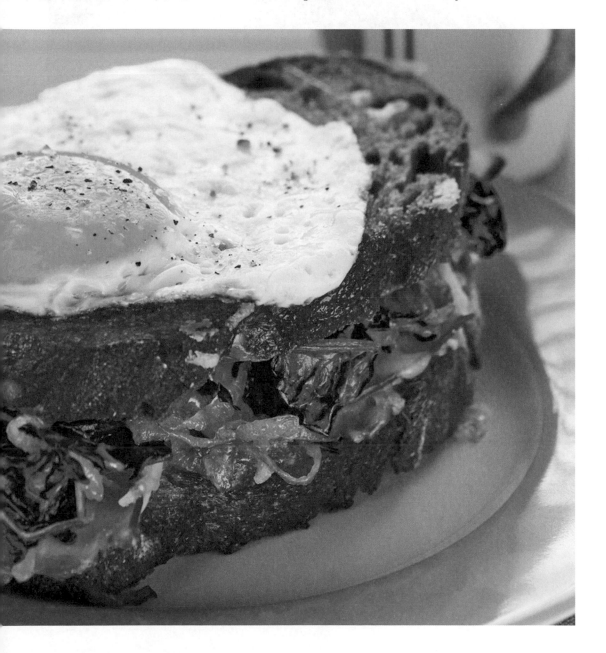

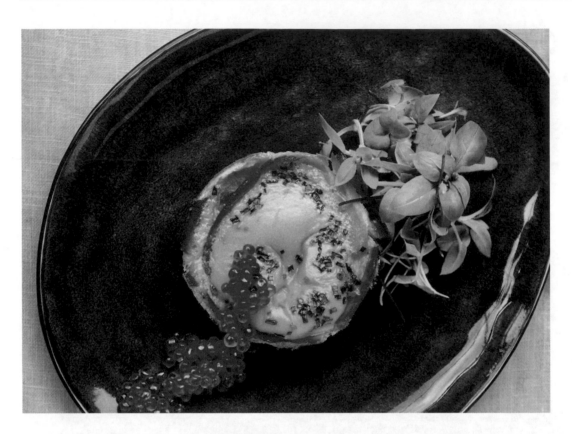

REFUELLING SALMON FRITTATAS

 SERVES 8 **CALS 87** **SAT FAT 2.2g** **READY IN 20 MIN**

WHY

Salmon and eggs are two of the best natural sources of omega-3, ideal after a workout because, according to studies, it fights muscle inflammation, helping you to recover quickly. Advice from the International Society of Sports Nutrition says if you're training hard, your protein requirements can be more than twice that of a normal person. Which we're taking to mean: have two.

INGREDIENTS

* **olive oil**, for greasing
* 8 slices of **smoked salmon**
* 8 **eggs**
* 50ml **milk**
* 1 tbsp chopped **chives**

METHOD

1/ Make sure you've got a muffin/cake tray ready for this. Now, preheat the oven to 200°C. Oil the tin and line each pocket with smoked salmon.
2/ Whisk the eggs and milk in a large bowl. Season, then add the chives. The next bit is easier if you pop this mixture into a jug, so you can pour it evenly into the eight muffin indentations.
3/ Place the tin in the oven and bake for 15 minutes, or until the frittatas are just set and are starting to go golden brown. Remove and leave to cool in the tin, then pop each one out and serve with some green leaves. Yep, we definitely want two.

ENERGISING NASI GORENG

SERVES **2** · CALS **290** · SAT FAT **7g** · READY IN **12**MIN

WHY

Broccoli and rice for breakfast? Hear us out. Brown rice is full of fibre, which slows down your digestion to keep you fuller for longer, while manganese and B vitamins in the broccoli release energy all the way through your Tabata class. "Coconut oil is a great source of medium-chain triglycerides, which studies show can increase energy expenditure and decrease body fat levels," says sports nutritionist Drew Price, author of *The Dodo Diet*. Beats Coco Pops.

INGREDIENTS

* 1 tbsp **coconut oil**
* 6 **spring onions**, sliced
* 1 **red chilli**, finely chopped
* 2 **garlic cloves**, finely chopped
* 1 tsp **garam masala powder**
* 200g **cooked brown rice**
* 100g **cooked broccoli**
* 1 tbsp chopped **fresh coriander**
* 2 **eggs**
* 1 tsp **white wine vinegar**
* 2 **lime wedges**
* **Sriracha chilli sauce**

METHOD

1/ Heat the oil in a large pan and fry the spring onions, chilli and garlic until softened. Then add the spices and cook for one more minute before adding the rice and broccoli.
2/ Cook for five minutes, then top with the coriander.
3/ Poach the eggs in boiling water and vinegar for three minutes. Serve the rice with an egg on top, drizzled with lime and chilli sauce for a spicy wake-up call. Hello hot stuff.

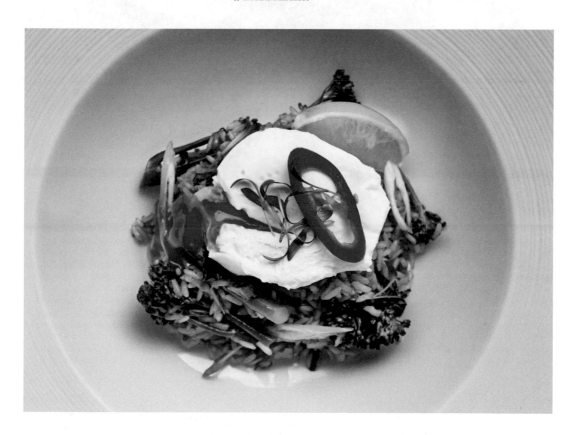

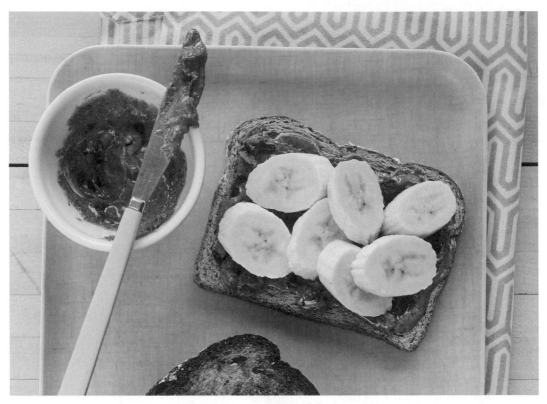

THE HEALTHIER ELVIS

SERVES **2** | CALS **418** | SAT FAT **2.5g** | READY IN **15**MIN

WHY

This breakfast option might look like something that made The King of Rock'n'Roll bust out of his jumpsuits, but it's actually an impressively healthy, morning-meal powerhouse. With meat *and* nut protein, potassium-rammed banana and slow-burn multigrain bread, you'll be sure of getting the energy you need to perform throughout the day. Uhhthangyewverrrmuch.

INGREDIENTS

 4 slices **multigrain bread**
 3 tsps **unsweetened almond butter**
 4 tsps crumbled, crisp-cooked **lean bacon**
 1 tsp **honey**
✹ ½ tsp **cinnamon**
✹ 1 large **banana**, sliced

METHOD

1/ Beat together the almond butter, bacon, honey and cinnamon in a small bowl. Divide this mix on two slices of bread, then spread evenly on each.
2/ Top both slices with sliced banana, then put the remaining slices on top. Sandwich with the remaining bread slices.
3/ Heat a large nonstick frying pan coated with cooking spray over a medium heat. Add the sandwiches and cook until golden and heated through, 4 to 5 minutes per side.

CARROT, BRAN AND CREAM-CHEESE MUFFINS

 MAKES **12** CALS **191** SAT FAT **3g** READY IN **40**MIN

WHY

See you later, muffin top – these baked goods will please your tongue and tum. The wholewheat flour, bran and flaxseed bring fibre which keeps you full for longer. And cinnamon has been shown to curb sugar cravings, too. Buttermilk (don't worry, it isn't made from butter) is rich in hunger-preventing protein, as well as vitamins A and C, which contribute to healthy, glowing skin. And there's even some carrots and raisins in the mix – not quite your five-a-day but they both bring antioxidants which slow down the ageing of cells – another bonus for your skin.

INGREDIENTS

* 90g **wholewheat flour**
* 100g wheat **bran**
* 170g ground **flaxseed**
* 100g **sugar**
* 1 1/2 tsps **cinnamon**
* 1 tsp **baking powder**
* 1/2 tsp **baking soda**
* 1 **egg**
* 250ml **buttermilk**
* 170g unsweetened **apple sauce**
* 2 **carrots**
* 70g flaked sweetened **coconut**
* 30g **raisins**

METHOD

1/ Heat the oven to 180°C and line a muffin tray with 12 paper cake cups.
2/ Whisk the flour, bran, flaxseed, sugar, cinnamon, baking powder, baking soda, and 1/2 tsp salt in a large bowl. In a separate bowl, mix the egg, buttermilk and apple sauce. Then stir the wet mixture into the dry ingredients and fold in the carrots, coconut and raisins. Spoon the batter equally between the paper cups.
3/ Bake the cakes for 30 minutes. Leave them to cool on rack, then top with cream cheese cinnamon spread: whisk 225g reduced-fat cream cheese, 3 tbsps honey, 1 tsp cinnamon, and 1/2 tsp vanilla extract.

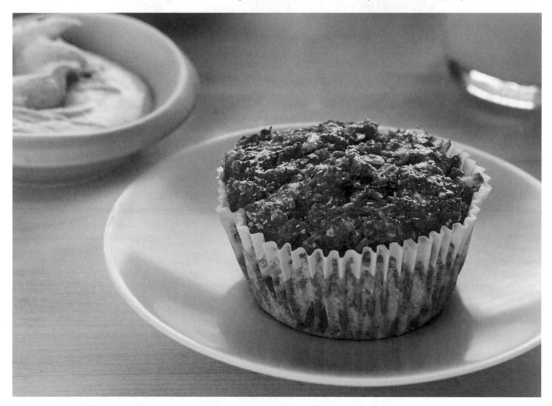

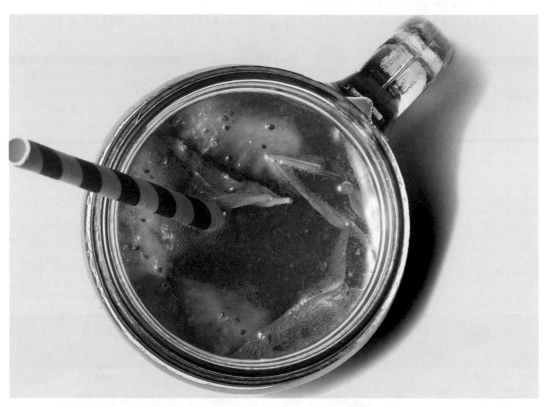

DE-STRESSING STRAWBERRY-ADE

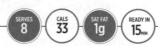

SERVES 8 · CALS 33 · SAT FAT 1g · READY IN 15 MIN

WHY

Had a long week? Verbena leaves contain essential oils to calm the nervous system and fight depression. And this will cheer you up: as well as being low GI for a slow release of energy, coconut palm nectar packs energising iron, heart-healthy potassium and B vitamins for glowing skin. The strawberries bring a sweet, fruity flavour, plus fibre and vitamin C. What's not to like?

INGREDIENTS

- 300g **strawberries**, sliced, plus a few extra for garnish
- 3 tbsps **coconut palm nectar**
- juice of 2 **lemons**
- 10g **lemon verbena leaves**

METHOD

1/ Put the strawberries, palm nectar and 250ml water in a pan. Gently warm for five minutes to dissolve the nectar, then remove the pan from the heat and leave to cool.
2/ Blitz the mixture in a food processor, then transfer it to a large water jug and add the lemon juice. Pour in 1 ½ litres of water and stir well before putting it in the fridge to chill for a couple of hours.
3/ Stir again, adding the lemon verbena leaves, a few extra sliced strawberries and some ice cubes to serve. Bottoms up!

BEAUTY-BOOSTING BAKED PANCAKE

SERVES **6** · CALS **155** · SAT FAT **0.5g** · READY IN **25** MIN

WHY

By cooking these pancakes in the oven, the frying part is skipped – saving you hundreds of oily calories (and possibly a blemish or two). The beauty-boosting properties are mostly from the buttermilk – it boasts a wealth of nutritional benefits including vitamins A and C, which bring a glow to the skin, and calcium, which strengthens your nails, teeth and hair.

INGREDIENTS

* 4 tsps **sugar**
* 120g **all-purpose flour**
* ½ tsp **baking powder**
* ¼ tsp **baking soda**
* 250ml **buttermilk**
* 4 tsps **vegetable oil**
* 1 **egg**
* ½ tsp pure **vanilla extract**
* **Icing sugar** (optional)
* 50g **mixed berries**
* 1 tbsp **lemon zest**
* 2 tbsps **sugar**

METHOD

1/ Heat the oven to 180°C. Mix the sugar, flour, baking powder, baking soda, and ¼ tsp salt in a large bowl. In a separate bowl, combine the buttermilk, oil, egg and vanilla extract, then stir into the dry ingredients.
2/ Lightly spritz a frying pan with cooking spray and add the pancake batter. Bake in the oven for 15 minutes, then remove and dust with icing sugar (optional).
3/ Cut and serve with berry compote: place 50g fresh mixed berries, 1 tbsp lemon zest and 2 tbsps sugar into a saucepan. Cook until berries soften, then lower the heat and cook for about 10 minutes, or until the sauce thickens (it'll be thinner than jam).

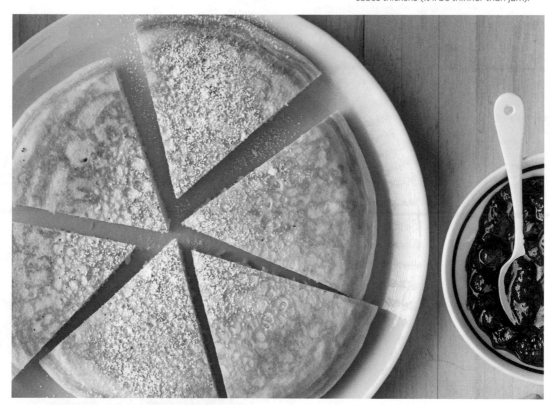

PHOTOGRAPHY: FRANCES JANISCH

SUPER

Here's a sweet swap – get glowing and boost your energy with fresh-tasting, customisable smoothies

SMOOTH

The seemingly virtuous smoothie has sunk to the level of health-food impostor – some bought concoctions pack more sugar than two doughnuts. We suggest these DIY alternatives: break out the blender and drink up

DETOX BEET-ORANGE BLISS

 SERVES **2**

 CALS **133**

 SAT FAT **0g**

 READY IN **10** MIN

Vitamin- and antioxidant-packed superfoods, including oranges, carrot juice and kale, help this dairy-free combo cleanse your system. Betalains in beetroot support your liver (the body's detoxification centre) for clear, glowing skin. Blend 120g chilled **green tea**, 80g **carrot juice**, 110g chopped cooked **beetroot**, 65g fresh chopped **kale** and 2 **oranges**, cut into segments and pith removed, in high-power blender and puree until smooth. Split between two glasses and sip away those toxins. Bliss!

PUMP UP THE PROTEIN
Throw in some shelled hemp seeds. And add some ground flaxseed for an extra dose of omega-3s.

SWITCH THE FLAVOUR
Try spinach or Swiss chard instead of kale; experiment with other citrus fruits, such as tangerine or pink grapefruit.

SERVES **2** **CALS** **98** **SAT FAT** **1g** **READY IN** **3** MIN

SUGAR SLASHING CHERRY-BERRY

This frothy 'milkshake' seems indulgent but is actually
a smart snack, thanks to the slow burn of low-GI strawberries
and cherries, while the protein in the yoghurt and skin-boosting
antioxidants in the fruit add a burst of nutritional goodness.
In your blender, pulse 120ml chilled **unsweetened almond milk**,
140g **plain**, **fat-free Greek yoghurt**, 255g **strawberries**,
250g **cherries** and 1-3 **ice cubes** until smooth.

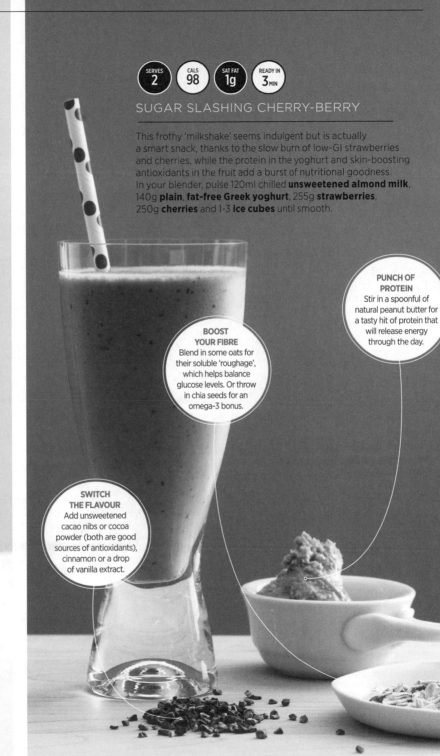

PUNCH OF PROTEIN
Stir in a spoonful of
natural peanut butter for
a tasty hit of protein that
will release energy
through the day.

BOOST YOUR FIBRE
Blend in some oats for
their soluble 'roughage',
which helps balance
glucose levels. Or throw
in chia seeds for an
omega-3 bonus.

SWITCH THE FLAVOUR
Add unsweetened
cacao nibs or cocoa
powder (both are good
sources of antioxidants),
cinnamon or a drop
of vanilla extract.

PHOTOGRAPHY: TINA RUPP

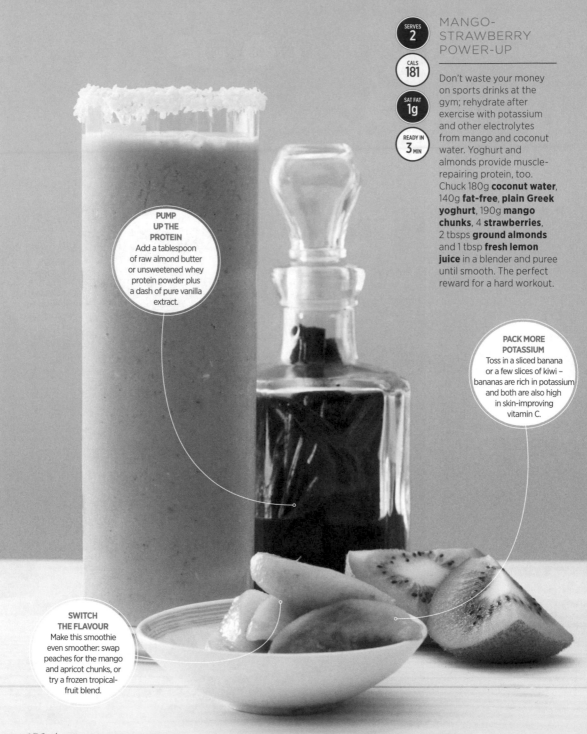

SERVES 2

CALS 181

SAT FAT 1g

READY IN 3 MIN

MANGO-STRAWBERRY POWER-UP

Don't waste your money on sports drinks at the gym; rehydrate after exercise with potassium and other electrolytes from mango and coconut water. Yoghurt and almonds provide muscle-repairing protein, too. Chuck 180g **coconut water**, 140g **fat-free, plain Greek yoghurt**, 190g **mango chunks**, 4 **strawberries**, 2 tbsps **ground almonds** and 1 tbsp **fresh lemon juice** in a blender and puree until smooth. The perfect reward for a hard workout.

PUMP UP THE PROTEIN
Add a tablespoon of raw almond butter or unsweetened whey protein powder plus a dash of pure vanilla extract.

PACK MORE POTASSIUM
Toss in a sliced banana or a few slices of kiwi – bananas are rich in potassium and both are also high in skin-improving vitamin C.

SWITCH THE FLAVOUR
Make this smoothie even smoother: swap peaches for the mango and apricot chunks, or try a frozen tropical-fruit blend.

SERVES **2** · CALS **221** · SAT FAT **1.5g** · READY IN **3** MIN

BANANA-AVOCADO ZINGER

Get a natural boost with energising B vitamins, which are found in foods such as bananas, avocado, spinach and parsley. The pineapple in this tropical blend provides manganese, a trace mineral that's essential for energy production. In your blender, blitz 120ml chilled **coconut water**, a **banana**, 1 small **avocado** (pitted, peeled and chopped), 15g **baby spinach leaves**, 120g **pineapple chunks**, 15g **fresh parsley** and 2 tbsps of **fresh lime juice** until smooth. How's your get-up-and-go now?

BOOST PROTEIN
Substitute the coconut water with skimmed or organic soya milk, or blend in unsweetened whey protein powder.

UP YOUR IRON
Use more spinach, parsley, leafy greens like mint or kale – or all of them – to get more of this energy-boosting mineral.

PICK UP THE PACE
Burn yourself out of snooze mode (well, sort of) with metabolism-stoking fresh jalapeño. Start with a pinch and adjust to taste.

PHOTOGRAPHY: TINA RUPP

POWER BLENDS

No time to cook? Here are 10 tasty blends, each bringing a burst of health-boosting nutrients to your body in minutes. Take your pick...

PEP-ME-UP VANILLA AND CINNAMON

Serves 2 | 111 cals
5g fibre

INGREDIENTS

❋ 1 **vanilla pod** ❋ 1 **banana**
❋ 250ml **almond milk** ❋ 1 tbsp
ground cinnamon ❋ 1 tbsp
hemp powder ❋ 4 **ice cubes**

METHOD

First, take a fresh vanilla pod. Cut off the ends and slice it lengthways to expose the seeds. Scrape a spoon along the length to collect them. Blend with the banana, and ice cubes. Knock back.
Juicy secret: Cinnamon has long been used in Chinese medicine to treat colds, indigestion and cramps. It also stabilises blood-sugar levels for a sweet kick that's far better for you than sugar.

PHOTOGRAPHY: STUDIO 33

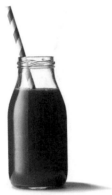

BRAIN-BOOSTING BEETROOT

Serves 2 | 237 cals | 16g fibre

✷ 1 bunch **organic raw beetroot**
✷ **3 organic cucumbers** ✷ **8 organic carrots** ✷ 200ml **water**

Blender ready? Keep any leaves on the beetroot as this is where a lot of the vitamins are stored. Oh, and don't peel the cucumber – its natural oils and collagen are in its skin. Chop the ingredients and blend, add the water and whizz till smooth. **Juicy secret:** Nitrates in beetroot increase oxygen flow to your brain. So that's your RDA of vitamin A, a source of iron and better concentration, all in one? Win.

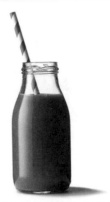

DETOXING SUPER GREEN

Serves 2 | 176 cals | 9g fibre

✷ **3 organic green apples** ✷ 250g **organic spinach** ✷ Small **bunch
parsley** ✷ **4 ice cubes** ✷ 250ml **filtered water**

There are green juices, and there are super-green juices. A lot depends on the quality of ingredients, so go organic if you can. Chop and core the apples, pop them in the blender and whizz up with the other ingredients. Simple. **Juicy secret:** Parsley is full of vitamins and is one of nature's best detoxing agents, helping to flush out toxins from the kidneys. The apples' sweetness takes the edge off its herby taste.

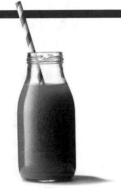

HYDRATING CELERY
AND SEAWEED

Serves 2 | 35 cals | 2g fibre

✷ 1 bunch **organic celery** ✷ 1 medium-sized **organic cucumber** ✷
squeeze **lemon juice** ✷ 2 tbsps **seaweed flakes** ✷ 250ml **filtered water**

Make sure the celery is firm. If it's wilted, sprinkle it with water and pop it in the fridge for a few hours to regain its crispness. Chop the veg and blend everything as usual – you're a pro by now. **Juicy secret:** Celery is the ultimate skin food. It's a whopping 95 per cent water, so it helps keep cells hydrated, plus it's full of vitamins A, B, C, K and folic acid, which support collagen production.

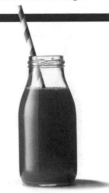

MEGA-HEALTH GINGER
AND CARROT

Serves 2 | 84 cals | 6g fibre

✷ **4 carrots** ✷ Juice of 1 **lime** ✷ 1/2 inch **knob ginger** ✷ 200g **spinach**
✷ Handful **parsley** ✷ 200ml **filtered water**

Peel and roughly chop the carrots. Pop them in the blender and whizz for a couple of seconds before adding all of the other ingredients. Blend, drink and soak up all that natural goodness. Mmm! **Juicy secret:** Ginger is one of nature's best all-round healers. It can help to clear sinuses, relieve nausea, ease joint pain and soothe stomach ache and bloating. Yep, it's a superfood alright.

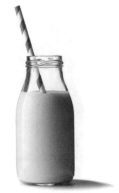

GERM-FIGHTING
COCO-CHOCOLATE

Serves 2 | 782 cals | 23g fibre

✱ 1 **coconut** ✱ 250ml **coconut water** ✱ 1 tbsp **raw, sugar-free organic almond butter** ✱ 1 tsp raw **cacao powder** ✱ 1 tsp **maca powder**

Crack open the coconut and scrape the insides into the blender. Throw in all the other ingredients and give it a whizz. Better than a Bounty! **Juicy secret:** Lauric acid in coconuts is a natural antibiotic, which can fight bad bacteria. It's also rich in caprylic acid, a potent antifungal to combat thrush and eczema. It has healing powers!

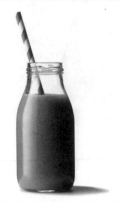

BLOAT-BUSTING DATE
AND COCONUT

Serves 2 | 208 cals | 7g fibre

✱ 1 **banana** ✱ 250ml **raw, unpasteurised coconut water** ✱ 4 **pitted dates**

The more ripe the banana, the better – unripe ones with blemish-free skins are less nutritious. Blend it with the coconut water until smooth, then throw in the dates and blitz again. Done. **Juicy secret:** Dates' sugars are slow-releasing, preventing the spike that could have you craving a Snickers an hour later. Cheers to that.

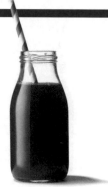

FLAT-BELLY BEET AND CARROT

Serves 2 | 221 cals | 13g fibre

✱ 4 **organic carrots** ✱ 1 bunch **organic beetroot** ✱ 2 **cucumbers** ✱ 1 **apple** ✱ 2cm **knob ginger** ✱ handful **mint** ✱ Juice 1 **lemon** ✱ 250ml **water**

Roughly chop the carrots, beetroot, apple and cucumbers. Add the other ingredients, blitz together in the blender and drink immediately. Just try not to spill it all over your fresh white T-shirt. **Juicy secret:** Mint leaves stimulate saliva production, warning your stomach to expect food, which aids digestion. Now that's handy when it has the roughage of the beetroot and carrots to deal with…

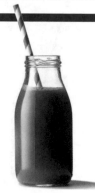

CLEANSING CUCUMBER AND MINT

Serves 2 | 186 cals | 12g fibre

✱ 2 **cucumbers** ✱ 1 **apple** ✱ handful **Swiss chard** ✱ 3 **mint leaves** ✱ 200g **alfalfa sprouts** ✱ 200ml **water** ✱ 1 tsp **chia seeds**

Whizz up the hard fruit and veg first (that's the cucumber and apple), then add the chard, mint, sprouts, water and seeds. Pick the smaller leaves of the chard because they taste less bitter. **Juicy secret:** Cucumber is a natural diuretic, speeding up your body's cleansing process to banish toxins. Natural oils in the skin also nourish and strengthen your hair, nails and skin. Definitely cool as.

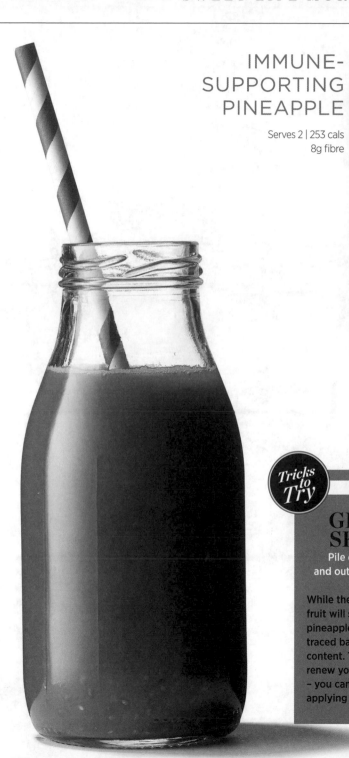

IMMUNE-SUPPORTING PINEAPPLE

Serves 2 | 253 cals
8g fibre

INGREDIENTS

✱ 4 **ice cubes** ✱ ½ **pineapple,** diced (including the core) ✱ 250ml **water** ✱ 2 **cucumbers** ✱ 250g **spinach** ✱ 1cm knob **ginger**

METHOD

If your blender has an ice setting, whizz the ice with the other ingredients to create a nice frothiness. If not, crush it in a tea towel with a rolling pin and add it at the end. For an optional extra kick, add a little grated ginger. Yum. **Juicy secret:** The pineapple core is rich in pain-relieving and anti-inflammatory bromelain. But it won't help if you get your hand stuck in the blender.

Tricks to Try

GET A SPIKY SKIN TREAT

Pile on the pineapple – inside and out – for smoother, clearer skin

While the usual antioxidants found in fruit will support skin production, pineapple's unique skin powers can be traced back to its hefty bromelain content. This enzyme won't only renew your complexion when eaten – you can supercharge the effects by applying the juice on the outside too.

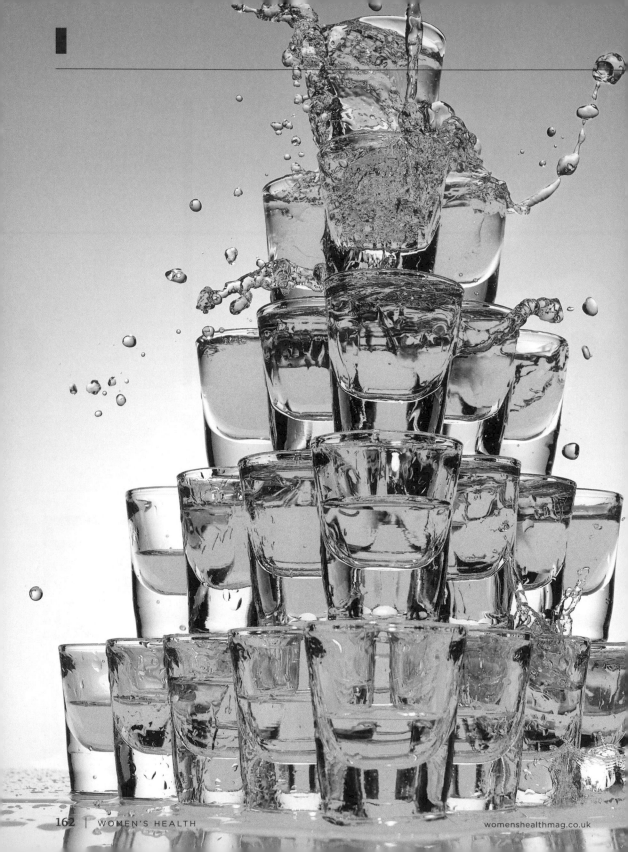

HEY, IT'S *SHOT O'CLOCK!*

How do you get the benefits of juice without the fibre-free, blood-sugar spike? We've found the answer

You're watching a group of twenty-somethings knock back shots at the bar – a little pick-me-up to stave off the effects from the night before. It's not a cheeky espresso or a horribly misguided tequila (life lesson: hair of the dog never wins in the end). It's called a 'wellness shot' or, as it's known by its street name, a very small juice. Yep, liquid devotees are downsizing. You may have noticed it at your local juice joint: fewer people chugging on 'venti'-sized cups of green gloop, while a new menu of smaller, cheaper alternatives is sprouting up.

Ed Foy spent five years living in the US before returning to Blighty to open Press*, the chic new addition to London's juice scene. And he's seen the trend spread across the pond. "Health-conscious Los Angelites were downing wheatgrass in the Nineties for a hit of vitamins and antioxidants," Foy says. "Cold-pressed wellness shots are a step from that."

And while they may have begun life in the world's wellness Mecca, Foy believes they found their foothold among the urban rush of New York – and now London. "Everyone is time-poor these days," Foy says. "They're not always looking for an indulgent drink – often, they want a quick solution."

And this is the USP of the juice shot. They're a medicinal tonic – downed to boost flagging energy, ward off a cold or settle a dodgy stomach. "People are turning against processed options – they'd rather consume something in its natural form than to take a synthetic vitamin," Foy adds. "The way shots are drunk, we can mix effective, curative ingredients like ginger, cayenne pepper and oregano oil. The taste isn't as important as they're going to be knocked back in one rather than sipped gradually."

But nutritionally speaking, do they have any benefit over longer juices? "In terms of vitamin absorption, smaller isn't necessarily any better," explains Rhaya Jordan, nutritionist at London juicing company The Juice Well. "Both are predigested – the fibre has been taken away, so the nutrients are absorbed as quickly as possible." The big win for shots is that they usually contain less fruit and sugar, because they don't need to taste as good. "For anyone wanting to avoid sugar, they're a good option," Jordan adds.

> "For anyone wanting to avoid sugar, they're a good option"

But how and when should you drink these dinky doses? It depends on why you're taking them. Knocking one back on an empty stomach, at least 15 minutes before eating, will ensure optimum absorption. But, Jordan says, swallowing straight after dinner means "the potent taste will turn on your saliva glands and kick-start digestion.

Either way, we've found the savviest shots to get you through your week – they're full of goodness and are definitely healthier than a tequila.

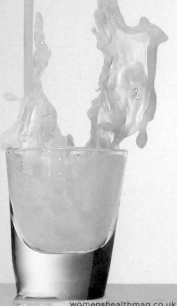

1

TAKE: Bee young shot by Juice Generation, NY*
WHEN: You feel groggy and grumpy in the morning.
HOW: Soak ¼ tsp bee pollen in 30ml coconut water for 10 minutes; strain before serving.
WHY: A study published in *Chemistry Central Journal* showed bee pollen has antioxidant properties, which can slow the ageing process. Totally buzzin'.

*PRESS (PRESS-LONDON.COM); JUICE GENERATION, NY (JUICEGENERATION.COM); THE JUICERY (THEJUICERYWORLD.COM); IMBIBERY (IMBIBERYLONDON.COM); THE JUICE WELL (THEJUICEWELL.

3

TAKE: Workout warm-up shot by Nosh Detox*
WHEN: Before you hit BodyPump.
HOW: Add 1 tsp turmeric and 1 tbsp liquid honey to a shot glass full of warm water. Simple.
WHY: The *Journal of the International Society of Sports Nutrition* revealed curcumin, found in turmeric, can prevent DOMS. Bring it on.

5

TAKE: Feel o-kale shot by The Juicery*
WHEN: Your dark-mornings SAD kicks in.
HOW: Blitz 40g pineapple, 20g kale and 8g ginger.
WHY: You need vitamin K from the kale to absorb dietary calcium – studies have linked this to helping prevent unstable moods.

2

TAKE: Hot flu-fighting shot by Imbibery*
WHEN: That itchy, scratchy throat starts.
HOW: Add half a piece of ginger to simmering water for 5-10 minutes before adding cumin seeds and a cinnamon stick. Bring the water to the boil and add paprika and cardamom.
WHY: The antiseptic properties of cumin can fight flu by boosting your immune system. Hot stuff.

4

TAKE: Tummy settlers shot by The Juice Well*
WHEN: You've got a food baby in your belly.
HOW: Blitz 15ml ginger juice and 5ml lemon juice with a pinch of cayenne pepper.
WHY: According to the University of Maryland, just 30mg of cayenne pepper three times daily can significantly reduce indigestion. Gut feeling.

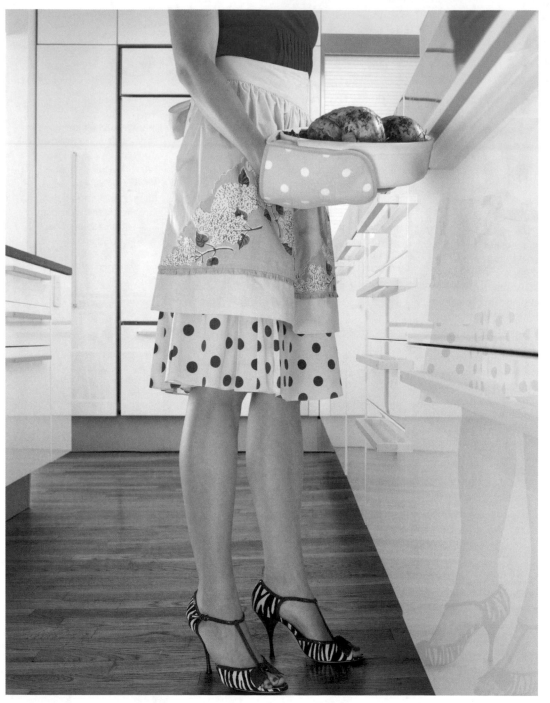

SWEET LIFE
MEALS

If you really want to enjoy the Sweet Life allowance of six tablespoons of added sugar a day, why waste any on hidden sugars in savoury meals? These delicious recipes, which range from quick-and-easy to luxurious slow-cook fare, are packed with energy-giving, metabolism-firing nutrients that will nourish your skin while you fill your face

BEAUTY BOOS

CITRUS AND GINGER SALAD

 SERVES **4** CALS **116** SAT FAT **2g** READY IN **10** MIN

WHY

This low-calorie lunch boasts over 200 per cent of your daily requirement of vitamin C – used by your body to produce collagen for softer, smoother skin. Tangerines and mandarins also contain nobiletin, a flavonoid compound which has been found to help prevent obesity. Team it with some quinoa or another nutty grain to bring on the zing in your lunchbox.

INGREDIENTS

* ✳ 2 **grapefruits**
* ✳ 2 **naval oranges**
* ✳ 3 **tangerines** (or 5 **mandarin oranges**)
* ✳ 1 tbsp **ginger**, chopped and crystalised
* ✳ 1 tbsp **pistachios**, chopped
* ✳ 2 tbsps **champagne vinegar**
* ✳ 2 tbsps extra-virgin **olive oil**
* ✳ **Mint leaves**
* ✳ **Salt**
* ✳ **Pepper**

METHOD

1/ Using a sharp chef's knife, chop the ends off each fruit. Then remove the skin and pith from the sides by moving the knife in a downwards motion, following the fruit's natural curve.
2/ Remove any white spots of pith you've missed, then cut the fruit into slices and arrange on a platter. Your very own work of art.
3/ Sprinkle on the ginger and pistachios, then drizzle with the vinegar and olive oil. Voila!

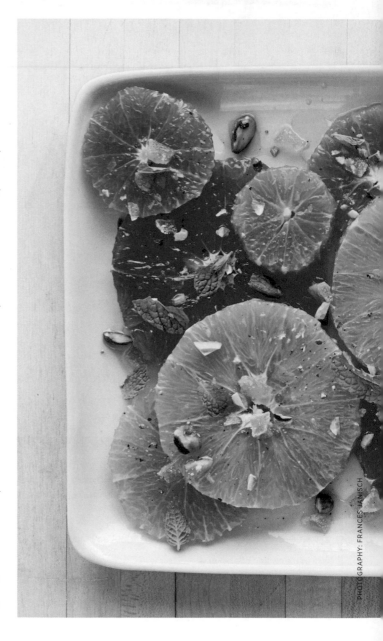

PHOTOGRAPHY: FRANCES JANISCH

TERS

Those ladies who lunch know something you don't! These clever, easy-to-prepare dishes will keep you full all afternoon, and give you glowing skin to boot

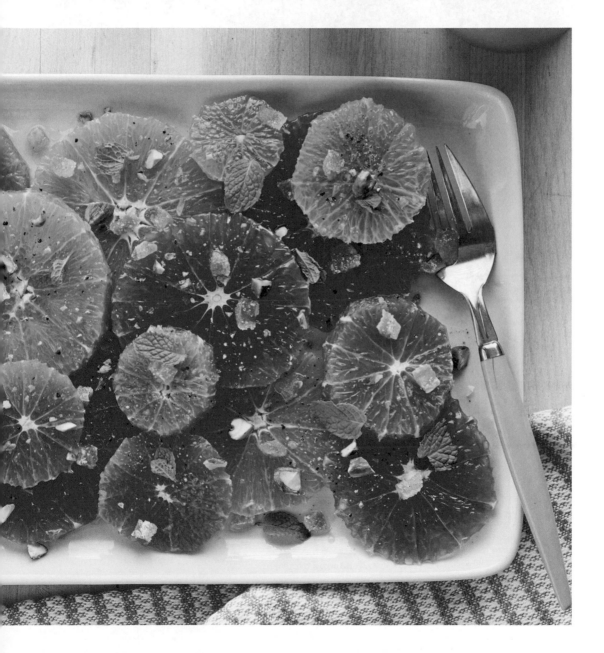

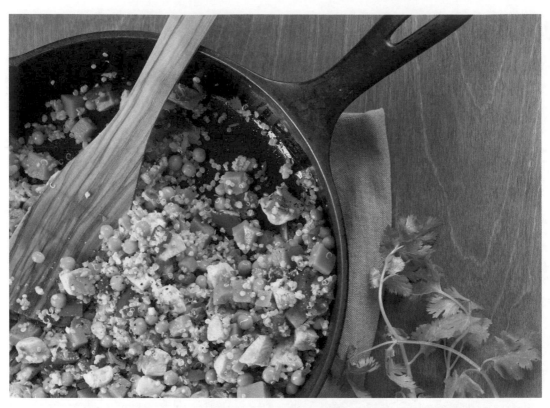

WRINKLE-FREE CHICKEN/SWEET-POTATO MIX

 SERVES 4 **CALS 307** **SAT FAT 1g** **READY IN 30 MIN**

WHY

The chicken and quinoa make an awesome team for hunger busting – the grain boasts twice the amount of protein as rice, so may well curb that 4pm chocolate-biscuit craving. And a study in the *American Journal of Clinical Nutrition* found that those who ate 100mg of vitamin C (half a sweet potato) every day for three years reduced the appearance of their wrinkles by 11 per cent. Cheaper than a facelift…

INGREDIENTS

* 180g cooked **quinoa**
* 1 **sweet potato**, peeled and cut into small cubes
* 4 tsps **canola oil**
* 340g boneless, skinless **chicken breast**, diced
* 1 **onion**, chopped
* 1 **jalapeño**, finely chopped
* 1 **red pepper**, chopped
* 1 **clove garlic**, crushed
* 1 tsp **ground cumin**
* 130g **frozen peas**
* 3 tbsps **coriander**, chopped

METHOD

1/ Simmer the quinoa in 250ml water, until all of the liquid has been soaked up.
2/ While your quinoa is doing its thing, boil the sweet potato until it's tender. Then drain the quinoa and sweet potatoes, separately.
3/ Heat 2 tsps of the oil in a non-stick frying pan. Add the chicken pieces and cook until they just start to brown. Empty into a bowl.
4/ Grab your frying pan again and add the remaining 2 tsps of oil. Stir in onion, jalapeño, red pepper, garlic and cumin. Cook for 3 minutes, then stir in the peas, chicken and cook another 2 minutes. Finally, stir in your quinoa and sweet potato and cook for 2 minutes. Garnish with the coriander. Boom.

PHOTOGRAPHY: MIKI DUISTERHOF

SPAGHETTI SQUASH PATTIES

SERVES **2** | CALS **354** | SAT FAT **3g** | READY IN **50** MIN

WHY

If you're fighting off the last of that lingering lurgy, then this is the recipe for you. Spaghetti squash (which, interestingly, can also be used as a great fill-in for pasta) is one of the best alkaline foods out there and is chock-full of antioxidant vitamins C and A. And it's those very antioxidants here that will leave your face feeling like it's been to a five-star spa, rather than the office kitchen.

INGREDIENTS

* 1 **spaghetti squash**
* 2 tbsps **sunflower oil**
* 1 **spring onion**, thinly sliced
* 30g finely chopped **leeks**
* 1⁄4 tsp **za'atar**
* 4g grated **ginger**
* 3g **coriander**, chopped
* 1 tsp **ground flaxseed**
* 1 tsp **ground coriander**
* 10g **oat flour**
* 3 tbsps **tahini**
* 5 tbsps **water**
* juice of 1 **lemon**

METHOD

1/ Heat the oven to 175°C. Cut the spaghetti squash in half, scoop out the seeds and drizzle with 1 tbsp oil. Bake for 40 minutes.
2/ Let it cool, then scoop out the insides with a fork. Put the strands into a large bowl.
3/ Add the spring onions to the squash with the leeks, za'atar, ginger, coriander, ground flaxseed and ground coriander. Mix with the oat flour and put it all into the fridge to cool.
4/ For the dressing, whisk the tahini, water and lemon juice with a fork. Nearly there!
5/ Heat the rest of the sunflower oil in a pan. When it's hot, make patties with the squash mixture. Sear until golden on each side. Serve with a salad and the dressing.

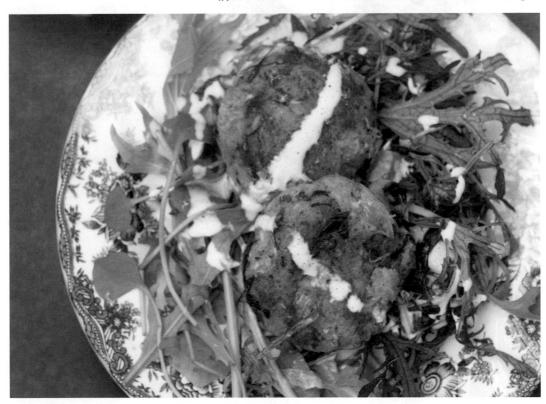

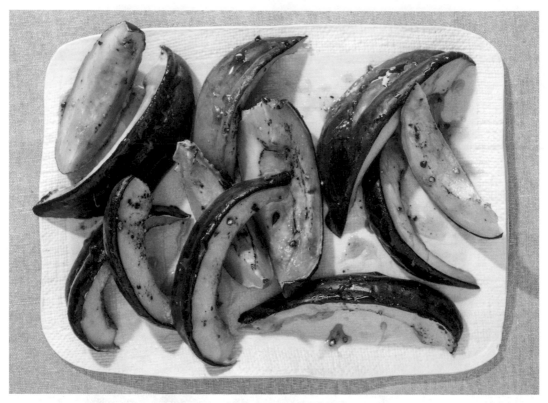

GLAZED BUTTERNUT SQUASH

 SERVES 4   **CALS** 240   **SAT FAT** 0g   **READY IN** 60 MIN

WHY

Alternative pub trivia for you: coconut sugar has 379 calories per 100g. The table variety has 1,700. The coconut kind is also much lower on the glycaemic index, so it's metabolised slower, avoiding that spike that has you stockpiling Curly Wurlys at 3pm. Made from the crystallised nectar of the tree's flowers, it also happens to be great at nourishing your skin – from the outside. When you're done with it in the kitchen, mix 1 tbsp with 2 tsps coconut oil for an all-natural body scrub that smells good enough to eat.

INGREDIENTS

✸ 250ml **pulp-free orange juice**
✸ 225g **coconut sugar**
✸ ½ tsp **cinnamon**
✸ 1 **squash**, halved and seeded

METHOD

1/ An easy job to start with – preheat your oven to 200°C. In a small saucepan over a medium to high heat, bring the orange juice to a boil. Reduce the heat to medium-low and add the coconut sugar and cinnamon. Simmer, stirring occasionally, until reduced by half (about 15 minutes).
2/ Place the squash, cut side up, in a baking dish. Pour 2 tbsps of the orange juice mixture into each half and baste the cut sides. Bake for 40 minutes, basting every 10 to 15 minutes. The squash should be golden and soft when done. It's a great accompaniment to the prawns, grilled chicken or fish. Sorted.

COCONUT CARROT SOUP

SERVES 4 — **CALS** 200 — **SAT FAT** 3g — **READY IN** 25 MIN

WHY

If your complexion is crying out for a little TLC, look no further than this soup, which is loaded with sources of the skin saviour beta-carotene (which improves both tone and texture) and zinging with spices and ginger, which contains over 40 antioxidant compounds that increase elasticity and boost circulation. And it's these spices that render the cocount water actually palatable, so you can enjoy all of the benefits without the love-it-or-hate-it-but-probably-hate-it taste getting in the way.

INGREDIENTS

* 1 tbsp **coconut oil**
* 450g **carrots**
* 1 **sweet potato**, peeled and chopped
* 1 **onion**, chopped
* 1 tbsp **ginger**, peeled and chopped
* 750ml **low-salt vegetable stock**
* 500ml **coconut water**
* 2 tbsps **lime juice**
* 1-2 tsps **curry powder**
* 1/4 tsp **ground cardamom**

METHOD

1/ Heat the oil in a pan over a medium heat. Now throw in the carrots, sweet potato and onion. Cover and cook, stirring occasionally, until softened.
2/ Add the ginger, stir and cook for 1 minute. Next, add the stock and bring to a boil, partially cover, then simmer for 10 minutes. Nearly there!
3/ Puree in a blender until smooth. Add the coconut water and blend. Return the soup to the pan, add the lime juice, curry powder and cardamom. Stir, then heat through. Garnish with red pepper, basil and spring onion, if desired. Now slurp.

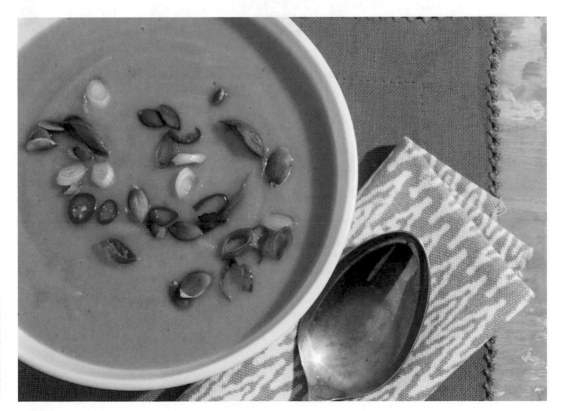

PHOTOGRAPHY: ZACH DESART

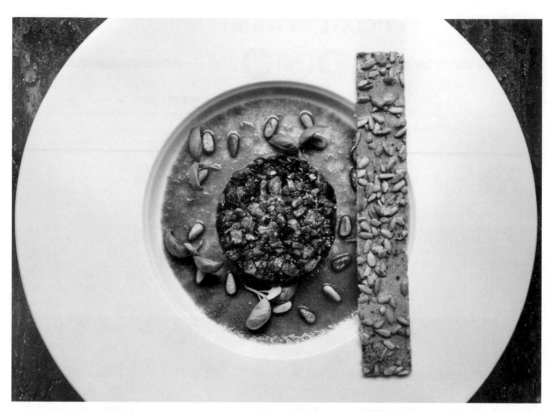

AUBERGINE CAVIAR WITH BASIL PISTOU

SERVES 6 · **CALS** 278 · **SAT FAT** 18g · **READY IN** 70 MIN

WHY

Treat your guests to a crowd-pleasing beauty cocktail with this impressive dish, which combines a bigger-than-usual quantity of basil with olives to create a powerful dose of antioxidants. Get this amazing variety of skin-renewing minerals from the aubergine (including copper, phosphorus and magnesium) and your own mother probably won't recognise you.

INGREDIENTS

* 3 large **aubergines**
* 350ml **extra-virgin olive oil**
* 4 tbsps **chopped Kalamata olives**
* 2 tbsps **pine nuts**
* 1 tbsp chopped **parsley**
* Zest and juice 1 **lemon**
* 380g **basil**
* 1 clove **garlic**
* 120ml **lemon juice**

METHOD

1/ Dice the aubergine then sauté it in 100ml olive oil until soft. Chill for an hour (the aubergine, not you).
2/ Mix with the chopped Kalamata olives, toasted pine nuts, parsley, zest and juice of the lemon and some sea salt and black pepper. Good work.
3/ Now for the pistou, a herby sauce. Whizz up the basil, garlic and lemon juice. Season and drizzle in the rest of the oil to form a green emulsion. Serve with the aubergine, toasted pine nuts, basil leaves and a seeded crispbread. Major domestic goddess points.

CHARD TARTAR WITH MACADAMIA CHEESE

SERVES 4 · CALS 831 · SAT FAT 13g · READY IN 150 MIN

WHY

Looking to give your skin a much-needed boost? You could smash up the piggy bank and make an appointment at the spa – or you could just cook up some chard. Rammed with brightening and renewing vitamins C and A and rich in plumping, smoothing omega-3, this leafy green is practically a makeover on a plate when teamed up with the nail and hair-building proteins of the macadamia nuts. Pretty tasty, eh?

INGREDIENTS

* 250g **macadamia nuts**
* 1.5 tbsps **vegan probiotic powder**
* 2 **shallots**, diced
* 380g **rainbow chard**
* 2 tbsps **sherry vinegar**
* 5 tbsps **olive oil**

METHOD

1/ Two days before your soirée, make 'cheese' with the macadamias. Cover the nuts in water and soak for 24 hours, then strain, keeping back the water. Add the probiotic to the water and whisk till frothy. Whizz this mix up with the nuts until smooth. Cover, then place in the fridge for 18-48 hours. Season and add shallots.

2/ Toss the chard in 2 tbsps of olive oil. Cover with foil and roast at 185°C for 2 hours. Peel, dice; pop in the fridge for 1 hr.

3/ Mix the sherry vinegar and the rest of the olive oil and drizzle over the chard. Serve with the cheese, and, if you like, add grapefruit, hazelnuts and micro amaranth.

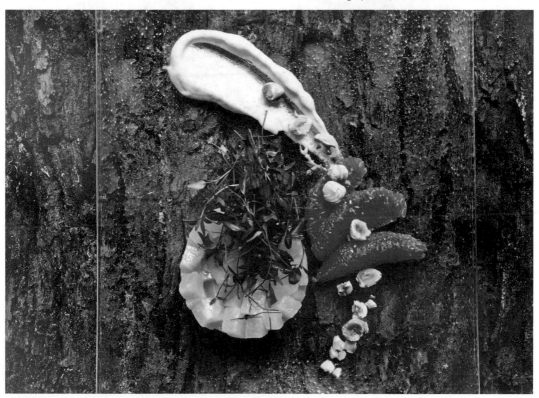

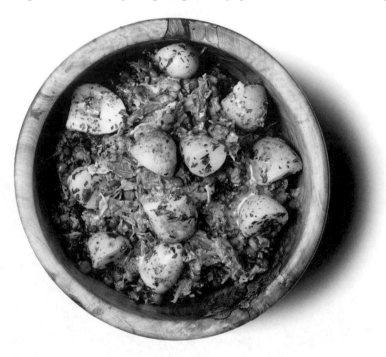

Perfect 10

SLOW-BURN SALADS

Leaves aren't just for summer. Michelin-star chef Marcus Wareing of Tredwell's restaurant shows you some more filling ways to enjoy their nutritional benefits

HEART-HEALTHY HAM HOCK SALAD

Serves 4 | 285 cals
2g sat fat | 25 mins

INGREDIENTS

✱ 320g **potatoes**
✱ 100ml **chicken stock**
✱ 320g **cooked ham hock**
✱ 300g **cooked lentils**
✱ ½ bunch of **parsley**, chopped
✱ cracked **black pepper**
✱ 1 tsp **Dijon mustard**
✱ 1 tbsp **grain mustard**
✱ 100ml **white-wine vinegar**
✱ 1 tbsp **honey**

METHOD

Start by chopping up the potatoes so that they're no larger than an egg, then boil them until cooked. Next, warm the stock in a large pan and add the ham. Cover and leave for 10 minutes, then stir in the lentils, parsley and pepper. Whisk the mustards, vinegar and honey together and drizzle over the potatoes and ham hock. Yummy.
Be-leaf it: Legumes like lentils can reduce your risk of heart disease, thanks to its fibre, folate and magnesium. Smart science.

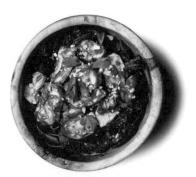

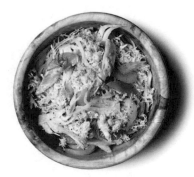

MOOD-ENHANCING CHICKEN & KALE

Serves 4 | 369 cals | 5g sat fat | 20 mins

✳ 2 **chicken breasts**, diced ✳ 5 tbsps **sesame oil** ✳ 5 tbsps **soy sauce** ✳ 1 tbsp **peanut butter** ✳ 500g **kale** ✳ 1 **red chilli**, chopped ✳ 1 tbsp **fish sauce** ✳ 50g **cashew nuts**, toasted ✳ ½ bunch **coriander**, chopped

Marinate the chicken in 1 tbsp sesame oil, 2 tbsps soy sauce and the peanut butter, then pan-fry until cooked. Heat 1 tbsp sesame oil in a wok. Wilt the kale with a pinch of salt. For a dressing, whisk 2 tbsps sesame oil and the remaining soy sauce with the chilli and fish sauce. Serve with the nuts and coriander. **Be-leaf it:** Folate in the kale boosts mood-regulating serotonin.

CRAB, FENNEL & PEAR MIX

Serves 4 | 288 cals | 5g sat fat | 15 mins

✳ 3 tbsps **extra-virgin olive oil** ✳ 300g **Dorset crab meat** ✳ Zest of ¼ **lemon** and 1 tsp juice ✳ 1 **large bulb fennel**, finely sliced ✳ 2 **ripe but firm pears** ✳ 25g **butter** ✳ 2 **star anises** ✳ 50g **frisee salad leaves**

Add one half of the olive oil to the crab with the lemon juice and zest, and the other half to the fennel. Peel and slice each pear into eight. Heat the butter and spices in a pan. Add the pears and roast until browned. Mix it all up and garnish with star anises and frisee. Easy. **Be-leaf it:** Crab has 19g protein per 100g, so this lunch will help you skip that 3pm biscuit.

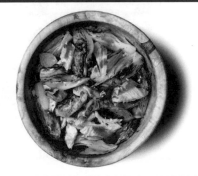

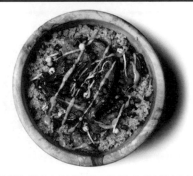

BRAIN-BOOSTING TROUT & LETTUCE

Serves 4 | 216 cals | 2g sat fat | 10 mins

✳ 320g **skinless smoked rainbow trout** ✳ 1 tbsp **vegetable oil** ✳ 4 **baby gem lettuces**, each cut into 3 wedges ✳ 50ml **chicken or vegetable stock** ✳ 50g **quince paste** ✳ ½ bunch **basil leaves**

Break the trout into chunks. Now heat the oil in a pan and brown the lettuce. Add a pinch of salt and stock and cook until it's tender. Heat the quince paste until it forms a glaze. Serve drizzled with the quince dressing; garnish with the basil. Bask in your cheffy glory. **Be-leaf it:** Rainbow trout has twice your RDA of omega-3, which boosts memory – hurray!

POST-GYM AUBERGINE & QUINOA

Serves 4 | 242 cals | 2g sat fat | 40 mins

✳ 2 **aubergines** ✳ 1 tbsp **harissa paste** ✳ 2 tbsps **vegetable oil** ✳ Juice of 1 **lemon** ✳ 2 tbsps **tahini** ✳ 1 tsp **smoked Tabasco** ✳ 1 tbsp **pomegranate molasses** ✳ 320g **cooked quinoa** ✳ 100g **sprouted beans** ✳ ½ bunch **parsley**, chopped ✳ 50g **pomegranate seeds**

Get that oven to 180˚C. Cut each aubergine into 16 strips. Cover in harissa paste, briefly fry in the oil, then bake until tender. Puree 8 of the strips. Whisk up the juice, tahini, Tabasco, molasses and salt, and drizzle over the quinoa, aubergine, puree, beans, parsley and pomegranate. **Be-leaf it:** Quinoa is a complete protein with all nine essential amino acids. Fab.

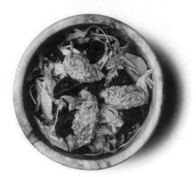

FLU-FIGHTING MACKEREL & BEETROOT

Serves 4 | 480 cals | 5g sat fat | 1 hour

✱ 16 **raw beetroots** ✱ 2 tbsps **walnut oil** ✱ 100g **low-fat ricotta** ✱ Zest of 1 **lemon** ✱ 2 tbsps **capers** ✱ 2 tbsps **tarragon** ✱ 1 tbsp **grain mustard** ✱ 320g **skinned smoked mackerel fillets** ✱ 100g **rocket**

Wrap 12 of the beetroots in foil; bake for 1 hour at 180˚C. Skin and chop them, then drizzle with oil. Peel and grate the other beets (wear gloves!). Mash with the ricotta, zest, capers, tarragon, mustard and salt and add the mackerel and rocket. **Be-leaf it:** Walnuts are rich in cold-fighting antioxidant polyphenol.

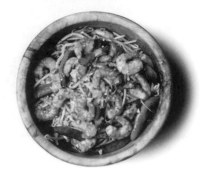

TUMMY-SOOTHING CHILLI PRAWNS

Serves 4 | 306 cals | 3g sat fat | 20 mins

✱ 2 tbsps **peanut butter** ✱ 2 tbsps **Sriracha** ✱ 1 tsp **fish sauce** ✱ 1 tbsp **soy sauce** ✱ 2 tbsps **vegetable oil** ✱ 350g raw, **peeled prawns** ✱ 200g **mangetout** ✱ ½ bunch **coriander**, chopped ✱ 50g **roasted peanuts**, finely chopped ✱ 100g **bean sprouts**

Whisk the peanut butter, Sriracha, fish sauce, soy sauce and 100ml water over a heat. Mix the prawns with the rest of the Sriracha and fry in 1 tbsp oil until pink. Heat the rest of the oil and chargrill the mangetout. Serve with coriander, nuts and bean sprouts. **Be-leaf it:** Coriander helps to ease upset tums.

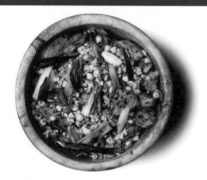

ANTI-INFLAMMATORY SWEET POTATO

Serves 4 | 333 cals | 2g sat fat | 45 mins

✱ 3 **sweet potatoes**, peeled ✱ 2 tbsps **vegetable oil** ✱ ½ **nutmeg**, grated ✱ ½ tsp **chilli flakes** ✱ 400g **tin chickpeas**, drained ✱ ½ bunch **coriander** ✱ juice and zest of 1 **lemon** ✱ 2 tbsps **extra-virgin olive oil** ✱ 3 tbsps **balsamic vinegar** ✱ 1 bunch **spring onions**

Coat the sweet potato with the oil, nutmeg, chilli and salt and bake for 25 mins at 180˚C. Mix the chickpeas with the coriander, juice and zest, olive oil and vinegar. Now char the onions and you're done. **Be-leaf it:** Sweet potato's anti-inflammatory quercetin can ease allergies and even asthma. As if we needed an excuse to eat wedges.

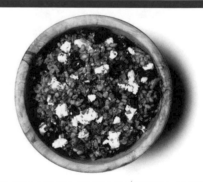

FLAT-BELLY BARLEY, PAPRIKA & FETA

Serves 4 | 471 cals | 7g sat fat | 30 mins

✱ 200g **pearl barley** ✱ 1 **onion**, sliced ✱ 1 **garlic clove**, crushed ✱ 1 tbsp **vegetable oil** ✱ 1 tbsp **smoked paprika** ✱ 2 tbsps **tomato puree** ✱ 50ml **extra-virgin olive oil** ✱ 100g **sunblush tomatoes** ✱ 50g **black olives** ✱ ½ bunch **parsley** ✱ 100g **feta**

Place the barley in a saucepan of cold water and bring to a gentle boil for 25 minutes. Fry the onion and garlic in the oil until golden. Mix in the paprika, tomato puree, olive oil, tomatoes, olives and some pepper. Pour over the barley. Top with the parsley and feta. **Be-leaf it:** Pearl barley has fewer calories than rice and twice the fibre. Guilt-free carbs *do* exist.

SKIN-LOVING BEEF & SQUASH

Serves 4 | 390 cals
8g sat fat | 30 mins

INGREDIENTS

* 1 **butternut squash**, peeled, seeded and cut into wedges
* 3 tbsps **vegetable oil**
* 350g **beef fillet tails**
* 25g **unsalted butter**
* ½ bunch **tarragon**, chopped
* 200g **mangetout**
* 50ml **balsamic vinegar**

METHOD

Preheat the oven to 180˚C. Brush the squash with 1 tbsp oil and a little salt. Bake for 20 minutes and set aside. Next up, brown the beef in a pan with 1 tbsp oil. Season, add the butter and baste for 5 mins. Coat the meat in the tarragon and allow to cool. Gently fry the mangetout in the remaining oil. Serve with the squash, beef and vinegar.
Be-leaf it: Betacarotene in butternut squash has skin-enhancing properties. Better than a sneaky lunchtime facial.

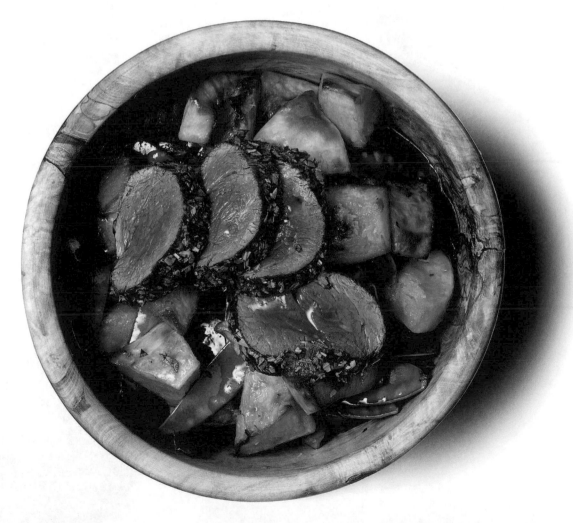

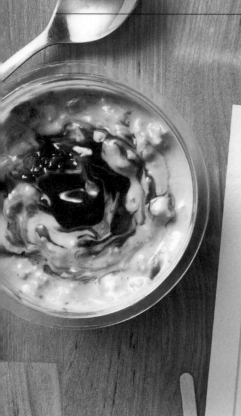

THE
COFFEE
— SHOP —

1 HOT DRINKS

Americano	£1.20
Espresso	£0.99
Hot Chocolate	£1.50
Mocha	£1.20
Cappuccino	£1.20
Tea	£0.99
Latte	£1.20

COLD DRINKS **2**

Iced Cappuccino	£1.50
Coffee Frappe	£2.25
Smoothie	£1.70
Iced Tea	£1.15
Bottled Water	£1.00
Orange Juice	£1.15

3 BREAKFAST

Egg & Bacon Sandwich	£3.50
Salmon & Egg Baguette	£3.50
Porridge	£2.00
Bircher Pot	£2.50
Ham & Cheese Croissant	£3.00

CAKES **4**

Salted Caramel Cake	£2.00
Almond Biscotti	£1.50
Bran Muffin	£2.25
Carrot Cake	£2.99
Millionaire's Shortbread	£2.50
Chocolate Chip Cookie	£1.5

THE *COFFEE* SHOP

When you're cutting sugar, here's a delicate middle ground to getting your café order right. Here's how you do it...

❶ HOT DRINKS

CHOOSE:
"At 20 calories, your best bet is an espresso," says nutritionist Amy Betts. "Or a flat white. Its 1:5 milk/coffee ratio means less fat than a latte." Cool beans.

LOSE:
Starbucks' hot chocolate has the same calories as two Crunchies. Cream on top is 150 more calories and 25 per cent of the UK recommended daily allowance of sugar.

❷ COLD DRINKS

CHOOSE:
A small iced cappuccino from Costa clocks in at 80 calories and 12.6g sugar. Or neck an iced Americano at Starbucks – it's just 11 calories. Very cool.

LOSE:
The strawberry and vanilla frappe at Caffè Nero. Tasty, yes, but at 470 calories and 54.4g sugar, it's actually the same as half a tub of Ben & Jerry's!

❸ BREAKFAST

CHOOSE:
A salmon and egg baguette. Pret's is just 320 calories and 1.6g sat fat, plus the salmon means you get some fat-burning omega-3s and protein. Yes!

LOSE:
"A bircher pot may seem healthy, but it's sugar heavy," Betts says. That's equal to an egg and bacon baguette in calories, and an extra 30g sugar. Oof.

❹ CAKES

CHOOSE:
Satisfy your sugar cravings with an almond biscotti, with around 150 calories, 1.5g saturated fat and 9g sugar. Perfect for guilt-free dunking.

LOSE:
The high-fibre bran muffin. The fibre is useful, but with an astonishing 23g sugar, you may as well go for a butter croissant with just 5.4g sugar. Oui, oui.

PHOTOGRAPHY: STUDIO 33

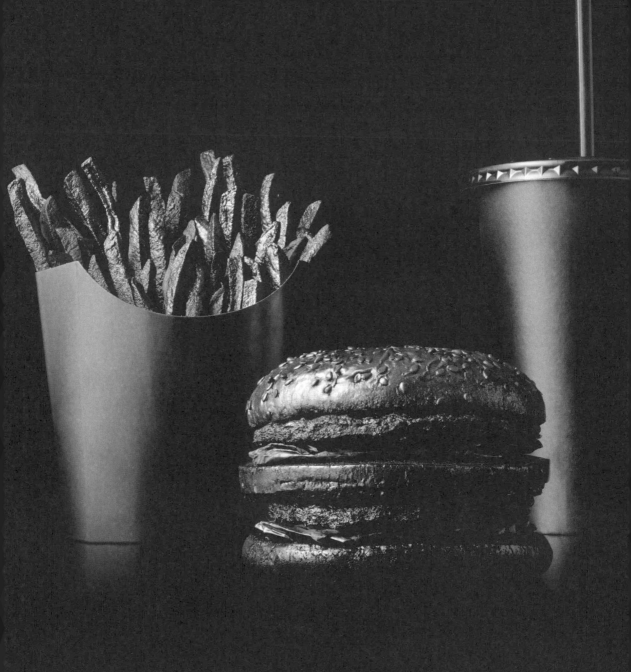

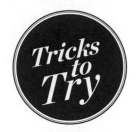

Tricks to Try

OUTWIT
TEMPTATION

Find it tougher to ignore sweet cravings (or any other kind) at certain times of day? You're not the only one – here's how to cheat them

Y ou've barely digested dinner, but you're already eyeing up that packet of biscuits like you're in the dying hours of a three-day juice fast. What's up? "Cravings are often blamed on dipping blood-sugar levels," says Dr Victoria Revell, chronobiologist at the University of Surrey. But it's not always the case. "Your circadian rhythm [body clock] also lowers your energy, leading you to crave high-calorie foods at certain times of the day." First step to not wolfing those calamitous cookies before bedtime? Identify your biological craving cause. Second step: use these strategies to beat it.

11AM MUNCHIES

"Two hours after breakfast, your blood-sugar levels will have dropped, making you hungry," says nutritionist Sarah Wilson, author of *I Quit Sugar for Life*. The bad news? According to a study in the *Journal of the American Dietetic Association*, women who ate mid-morning lost less weight and tended to carry on picking throughout the day. Step, away.

THE SWERVE: Get this: snack avoidance begins at breakfast time – and we've already explained how. Researchers in Louisiana, US, found that people who started their day with an egg had lower levels of the appetite-stimulating hormone ghrelin three hours later than those who started their day with cereal. Absolutely need a snack? Go for almonds – in a US study, people who ate 43g of them (250 calories worth) as a mid-morning snack were so satiated that they consumed fewer daily calories overall. Snack win.

3PM SLUMP

That afternoon slump can be avoided by swerving a carby lunch, right? Not entirely true. "Your body's circadian rhythms lead to a dip in energy levels after lunch, that can occur whatever you eat," Revell says. "This may be linked to a natural inclination for sleep every 8-12 hours." But when napping isn't an option, your brain seeks a nutritional energy boost: sugar!

THE SWERVE: A University of Wyoming study found that an hour of moderate cardio at lunch can quash your appetite for the next two hours – if you stay hydrated. Meanwhile, your energy dip may be compounded by a drop in mood-boosting serotonin. "Your brain needs carbs to produce serotonin," explains Dr Judith Wurtman, author of *The Serotonin Power Diet*. "You need around 30g of carbs for that quick serotonin lift." Think a wholemeal bread roll, a banana or 50g dried apricots. Nibble away. Then stop.

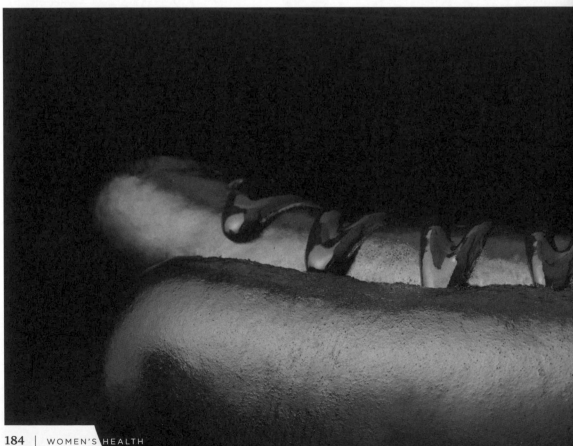

10PM BINGE

It's not just that painful episode of *Don't Tell the Bride* sending you to the fridge: a study in the journal *Obesity* found we may be programmed to crave sweet, high-cal foods at night. "This tactic might have helped our ancestors when food was scarce," Revell says. "Eating before sleep meant they stored the calories more efficiently." Problem? You're not a caveman. **THE SWERVE:** "Your body doesn't metabolise food as well at night, so avoid munching," Revell says. Try this trick to deal with cravings: "Take two teaspoons of coconut oil," Wilson says. "It's made up of medium-chain fatty acids (MCFAs), which deliver quick energy to your body, without producing an insulin spike in your bloodstream." You can eat it straight from the jar, but for a more palatable option, pop a couple of teaspoons in some warm almond milk and sweeten with cinnamon. Cheers!

4AM FREAK OUT

Terrorist threats, overdraft limits, the impact of climate change on the global goji berry harvest… It's enough to keep you awake at night. But that early morning panic attack may not just be down to stress. "If you wake abruptly in the early hours, it may be the result of something called nocturnal hypoglycaemia," women's health expert Dr Marilyn Glenville says. "It's caused by your blood sugar dropping – your body releases adrenaline to correct the imbalance, and that wakes you up." **THE SWERVE:** Easy. "Have a protein-rich evening meal with minimal starchy carbs," Glenville says. "Try grilled fish and veg. Then, about an hour before bed, have a small complex-carb snack, such as an oatcake or half a slice of rye bread. This will stop your blood sugar dropping during the night." And you'll be less worried about the poor goji berries.

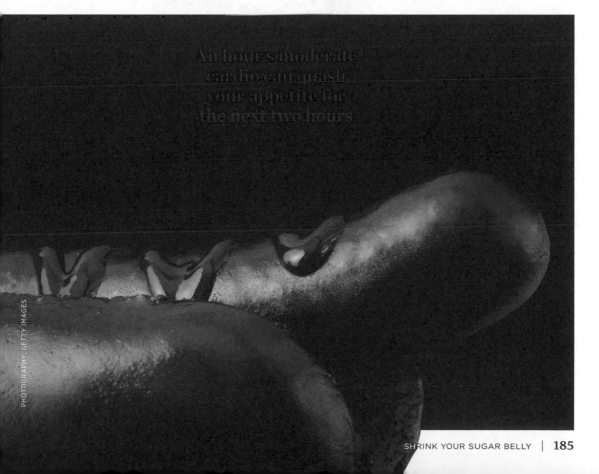

An hour's moderate cardio can quash your appetite for the next two hours

PHOTOGRAPHY: GETTY IMAGES

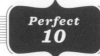

Perfect 10

SLIM-TUM TAPAS

We love a big, spicy chorizo as much as the next girl, but diet-friendly,
it ain't. Here's a lighter, more nutritious take on Spanish finger food

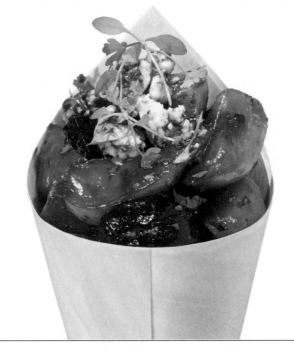

LOVE-ME-TENDER BEETROOT

Serves 4 | 384 cals
7g sat fat | 40 mins

INGREDIENTS

* ✷ 600g **baby red and yellow beetroots**, leaves cut off
* ✷ Handful of **table salt**
* ✷ 100g best-quality **blanched hazelnuts**, roughly chopped
* ✷ 50ml **extra-virgin olive oil**
* ✷ 15ml **hazelnut oil**
* ✷ 4 tbsps **fresh chives**, chopped
* ✷ 25ml **moscatel vinegar**

METHOD

Place the baby beets (cute) in a large pan with the table salt. Cover with cold water, bring to the boil and cook until tender – around 20 to 30 minutes. When the beetroots have cooled, peel them and slice into rounds. Mix the remaining ingredients in a bowl and pile the beetroots into the dressing. **Bite size:** Beetroot increases blood flow and sends oxygen to your noggin. Consume pre-Trivial Pursuit for the full benefit.

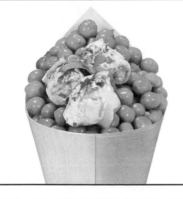

PEAS-AT-LAST WITH QUAIL EGG

Serves 4 | 261 cals | 2g sat fat | 10 mins

✳ 2 large **shallots**, peeled and finely diced ✳ 2 **garlic cloves**, finely chopped ✳ 200ml **chicken stock** ✳ 20g **unsalted butter** ✳ 8 fresh **mint leaves**, finely sliced ✳ 400g **fresh peas**, shelled and blanched ✳ 400g **broad beans**, shelled and blanched ✳ 1 **quail egg**, poached

Fry the shallots and garlic for 3 minutes in oil. Add the stock and bring to the boil. Simmer for 5 minutes, add the butter, mint, peas and beans; simmer for 2 minutes. Serve with the poached quail egg. **Bite size:** Broad beans boast more fibre than broadband which helps your cardiovascular health!

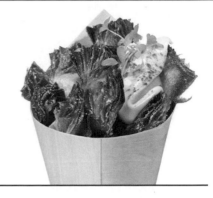

GET-IN-ME CONFIT ARTICHOKES

Serves 4 | 269 cals | 1g sat fat | 45 mins

✳ 1.5 litres **olive oil** ✳ 2 **carrots**, peeled and diced ✳ 1 **leek**, finely diced ✳ 2 heads of **garlic**, halved horizontally and roasted ✳ Bunch **fresh thyme** ✳ 4 **bay leaves** ✳ 20 **baby artichokes**, trimmed and peeled ✳ **Lemon juice** ✳ **Aioli**, enough to dip

Heat the oil and add the carrots, leek, garlic and herbs. Add the artichokes and cook for 25 minutes. Drain, discard the other veg and place the stalk upwards to drain off any excess oil. Squeeze the lemon juice over the aioli and dip away. **Bite size:** An artichoke packs nine times more vit C than orange juice.

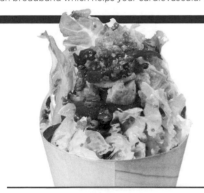

CATCH-A-BITE TUNA SALAD

Serves 4 | 215 cals | 3.5g sat fat | 10 mins

✳ 200g **ventresca tuna fillets** ✳ 1 **shallot**, peeled and diced ✳ 5ml **sherry vinegar** ✳ 15ml **olive oil** ✳ 2 tsps **fresh chives**, chopped ✳ **Salt** and **pepper** ✳ 4 baby gem lettuces, quartered lengthways ✳ 4 **piquillo peppers** ✳ Handful fresh **flat-leaf parsley**, chopped

Pop the tuna on the grill. Mix the shallot, vinegar, oil and chives and season with salt and pepper. Arrange the baby gem on a serving dish and spoon over the dressing. Top with the tuna, peppers and parsley. **Bite size:** Ventresca tuna is a great source of immune-boosting selenium and vitamin D.

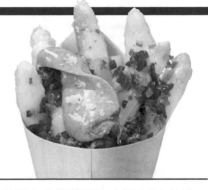

WELL-DRESSED ASPARAGUS

Serves 4 | 283 cals | 3.75g sat fat | 35 mins

1 **sweet piquillo pepper** ✳ ½ tsp **green pepper** ✳ 1 **shallot** ✳ 1 bunch **chives**; 1 **prawn**, cooked ✳ 150ml **olive oil** ✳ 50ml **sherry vinegar** ✳ ½ tsp **smoked paprika** ✳ 1 **egg yolk** ✳ 700ml **olive oil** ✳ 100ml **warm water** ✳ 1 **lemon**, juiced ✳ 60ml **vinegar** ✳ 1 **orange**, juiced ✳ 12 large **white asparagus**, blanched ✳ 1 **egg**, boiled

Chop the peppers, shallots and chives, and mix with the oil, vinegar and spice. Whisk the yolk and oil until you have a thick mayo. Stir in the remaining ingredients. Top the asparagus with the dressing, mayo and grated egg. **Bite size:** Cheeky asparagus boosts collagen and reduces the appearance of fine lines.

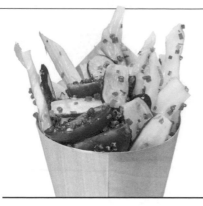

CHUCK-TOGETHER FENNEL SALAD

Serves 4 | 290 cals | 4g sat fat | 10 mins

✸ 80g **black radishes** ✸ 16 **red radishes** ✸ 1 **bulb fennel** ✸ 8 tbsps **olive oil** ✸ 4 tbsps **moscatel vinegar** ✸ 4 heads **red chicory**, base trimmed and leaves off ✸ 4 tbsps **fresh tarragon**, chopped

Whip out your mandolin (slicer) and slice the radishes and the fennel. Whisk the olive oil and vinegar. Add the radishes, fennel, chicory and tarragon, season and mix well. *Buen apetito*! **Bite size:** The most potent bulb since the LED, fennel is rich in anethole which has been shown to prevent cancer.

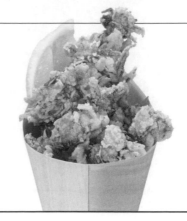

THE SUNDANCE SQUID

Serves 4 | 542 cals | 4g sat fat | 15 mins

✸ 1 litre **oil** ✸ 200g ground **Andalusian flour** (or mix 100g **plain flour** and 100g fine **breadcrumbs**) ✸ 450g **baby squid**, cleaned ✸ 1 **garlic clove**, peeled and finely chopped ✸ 1 tsp **fresh thyme leaves** ✸ 1 **lemon**, quartered

Heat the oil in a large pan. Put the flour in a bowl and toss through the squid, coating them well. Fry for 3 minutes, until crisp, then drain them on a paper towel. Serve with garlic, thyme, pepper, salt and lemon. **Bite size:** Lemon aids digestion by neutralising toxins in the stomach. Sharp one.

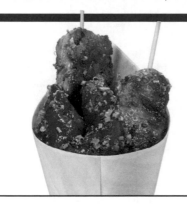

HOT-HOG SKEWERS

Serves 4 | 562 cals | 8.6g sat fat | 80 mins

✸ 400g **lean pork fillet**, diced ✸ 4 **cloves garlic**, crushed ✸ 200ml extra-virgin **olive oil** ✸ **Spice mix** (10g **ground cumin**, 10g **smoked paprika**, 10g **oregano**) ✸ 8 **sweet preserved piquillo peppers** ✸ 4 **bay leaves**

Marinate the pork in the garlic, olive oil, spice mix, piquillo peppers and bay leaves. Skewer the meat and peppers onto 4 sticks and grill on a high heat for 30 seconds on each side, turning three times. **Bite size:** Cumin and oregano are rich in iron. Ideal for those fighting low moods. Smile, now.

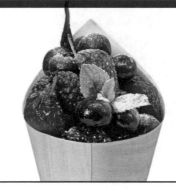

MERRY BERRY SALAD

Serves 4 | 293 cals | 3.2g sat fat | 10 mins

✸ 150g **blueberries** ✸ 150g **raspberries** ✸ 150g **strawberries**, sliced ✸ 2 tbsps **xylitol** ✸ 8 **mint leaves** ✸ 4 tbsps **olive oil** ✸ 1 tsp **sherry vinegar** ✸ 2 **limes**, juiced ✸ 1 **vanilla pod**, split lengthways ✸ 1 bunch **fresh oregano**

Mix the oil, vinegar, limes, vanilla pod and marjoram, and pop in the fridge for 24 hours. Next day, divide the fruit into bowls and sprinkle with xylitol. Remove the vanilla pod and oregano from the dressing, drizzle over the fruit and garnish with mint. **Bite size:** Small doses of oregano calm stress levels.

RING-A-DING-DING CUTTLEFISH

Serves 4 | 560 cals
6.4g sat fat | 50 mins

INGREDIENTS

* ✱ 240g **cuttlefish**, sliced into rings
* ✱ 12 tbsps **olive oil**
* ✱ 1 large **shallot**, chopped
* ✱ 500ml **chicken stock**
* ✱ 240g **dried chickpeas**, boiled and drained with one onion
* ✱ 300g **baby spinach leaves**
* ✱ **Seasoning**
* ✱ 4 **ice cubes**

METHOD

Brown the cuttlefish in hot oil. Then add the shallots for 2 minutes. Add the stock to the pan and simmer until it has reduced by half. Add the chickpeas and simmer for 5 minutes, then the spinach for a further 30 seconds. Drizzle with olive oil and season. **Bite size:** Spinach has potassium (more than bananas) and magnesium – both great for a healthy metabolism. A tapas HIIT!

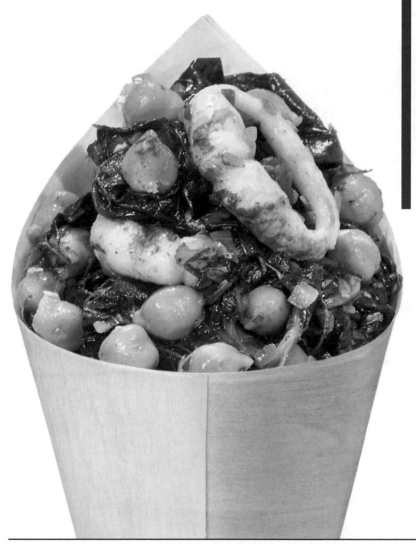

INDIAN 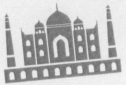 CUISINE

STARTERS
MULLIGATAWNY
£2.95

DHAL SOUP
£2.95

ONION BHAJI
£2.95

VEGETABLE SAMOSA
£2.95

VEGETABLE PAKORA
£2.95

CHICKEN PAKORA
£3.95

CHANA PURI
£2.95

MAINS
TANDOORI CHICKEN
£6.95

CHICKEN MADRAS
£6.95

BEEF VINDALOO
£6.95

CHICKEN JALFREZI
£7.50

SAAG CHICKEN
£7.50

LAMB BHUNA
£7.50

CHICKEN KORMA
£7.50

CHICKEN KASHMIRI
£7.50

LAMB ROGAN JOSH
£7.50

LAMB PASANDA
£7.50

SIDES
PILAU RICE
£1.95

KEEMA PILAU RICE
£2.95

MATTAR PILAU RICE
£2.50

BOILED RICE
£1.95

FRIED RICE
£2.50

EGG FRIED RICE
£2.95

SAFFRON RICE
£2.95

CHAPATI
£1.90

PLAIN NAAN
£1.90

PESHWARI NAAN
£2

THE *INDIAN* RESTAURANT

*Kicking out cravings with spice is a valid sugar-belly strategy –
just make sure you steer clear of these fat traps while you do it*

❶ STARTERS

CHOOSE:

A broth-based mulligatawny or dhal soup has 150 fewer calories than one onion bhaji. Plus, a Penn State University study found starting with soup resulted in 20 per cent fewer calories eaten afterwards.

LOSE:

Bhajis, samosas, pakoras and purees all begin life in the deep-fat fryer. At 200 calories a pop and with around 10g of fat in each, avoid them at all costs.

❸ RICE

CHOOSE:

A good low-fat choice is saffron rice, with just 0.5g fat and 335 calories per serving.

LOSE:

"Rice with veg [pilau or biryani], boosts your vitamin intake but adds fat as they tend to be cooked in more oil," says dietician Azmina Govindji.

❷ MAIN DISHES

CHOOSE:

Veggie or meat bhuna, jalfrezi or rogan josh are your best bets. The sauce is reduced and the tomato base means the damage is limited to 350 calories and 20g fat.

LOSE:

Makhani, korma, pasanda and masala curries involve cream, ghee (clarified butter) or khopre (coconut oil), with 800 calories and more than 40g fat. Swerve.

❹ SIDES

CHOOSE:

Go for the chapati. Ghee-free, you'll get around 110 calories and 0.5g fat per chapati slice. Add on 70 calories if dipping in mango chutney.

LOSE:

The average naan sneaks in 540 calories (which shoots up to 700 if you go for the peshwari variety) and a whopping 20g of fat. Naanbelievable.

PHOTOGRAPHY: STUDIO 33

HIGH-ENERGY

COCONUT LIME TILAPIA FISH

 SERVES 4 **CALS** 230 **SAT FAT** 8g **READY IN** 15MIN

WHY

Team the iron-rich spinach with easily-digested delicate protein of the tilapia fish and you've got yourself a slow-burn, energy-rich dish which won't slow you down to digest. The benefits of cooking with coconut oil go from the sublime (better skin, a smaller waistline) to the ridiculous (reduced risk of baldness – yes, really).

INGREDIENTS

* ✳ Zest of 3 **limes**
* ✳ 4 cloves **garlic**, crushed
* ✳ 5 tbsps **coconut oil**, melted
* ✳ 4 x 150g **tilapia fillets**
* ✳ fresh **spinach**
* ✳ 1 tbsp **lime juice**

METHOD

1/ Heat a large, non-stick frying pan over a medium-high heat. In a small bowl, mix up the lime zest, garlic, salt, pepper and 4 tsps of coconut oil.
2/ Coat the tilapia fillets with the oil mixture on both sides. Place them, two at a time, in the pan and cook for 4 minutes on each side, until golden and crisp. Smells good, right?
3/ In a large bowl, toss the spinach with the remaining 1 tbsp coconut oil and 1 tbsp lime juice. Divide among four serving plates. Serve each fillet on top and drizzle with extra lime juice. Hold back on the chips, though.

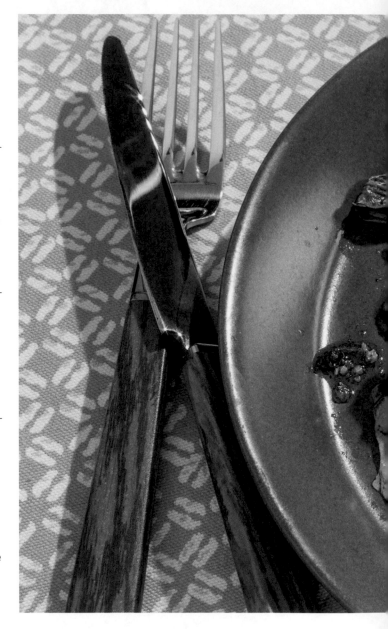

EATS

It's time to fend off your post-meal slumps with these impressive dinner dishes

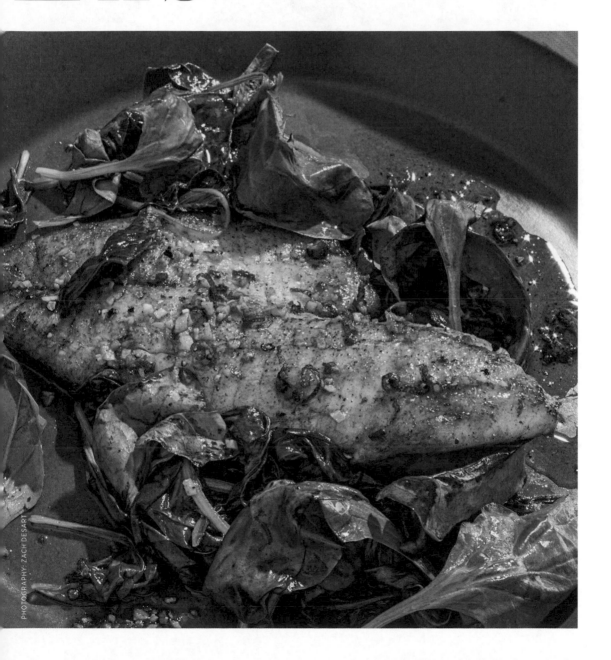

PHOTOGRAPHY: ZACH DESART

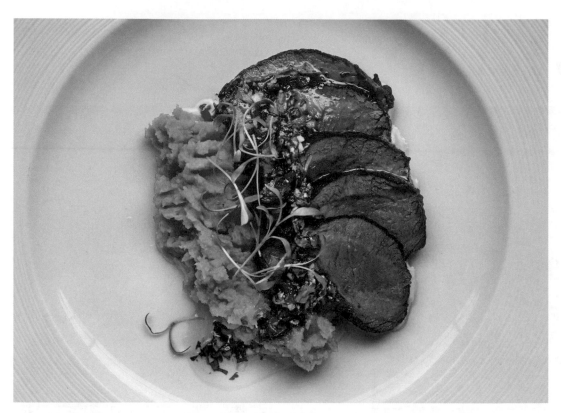

BODY-BUILDING VENISON WITH SWEET POTATO

SERVES **4** | CALS **52** | SAT FAT **27g** | READY IN **70**MIN

WHY

You probably know your muscles need a protein injection to help them repair after workouts, but did you know how good venison is for this? It's lower in fat than chicken, higher in iron than beef and is organic and wild. Plus, it's higher in omega-3, which increases feelings of fullness so you (probably) won't want dessert. If all that wasn't enough, tryptophan in the sweet potatoes helps to convert the venison's protein into serotonin, the hormone that'll guarantee you a decent night's sleep. Talk about a winning evening-meal combo.

INGREDIENTS

✳ 600g **sweet potatoes**, diced
✳ 4 x 200g **venison steaks**
✳ 1 **red chilli**, chopped
✳ 1 small handful **coriander**
✳ 1 tbsp **cider vinegar**
✳ 1 tsp **honey**
✳ 150ml **olive oil**

METHOD

1/ Kick things off with the sweet potato by putting it in a saucepan with salted water. Boil, then reduce the heat and simmer, covered, for 20 minutes. Drain and mash 'em with a little salt and pepper.
2/ Meanwhile, heat a ridged griddle pan and season the steaks generously. Cook, turning them over often, for 10 minutes until browned with a little pink in the middle.
3/ Let the venison rest for five minutes before slicing. While it's resting, rustle up the dressing by blending the chilli, coriander, vinegar, honey and olive oil.
4/ Drizzle the dressing over the steaks and serve with the sweet-potato mash!

PHOTOGRAPHY: NATO WELTON

PROTEIN-POWER GLAZED PORK WITH SUCCOTASH

 SERVES **4** CALS **251** SAT FAT **1g** READY IN **30**MIN

WHY

Who said pork is unhealthy? Well, covered in oil in a fry-up, yes – but if you opt for a lean cut, such as tenderloin, and remove all the visible fat, you're left with a pretty nutritious piece of meat. Pork is high in protein, which helps to keep you full and also speeds up muscle growth and repair (gym bunnies, rejoice). Okra is rich in vitamin A, which helps vision and keeps your skin nice and healthy. And cider vinegar? It's been shown to aid weight loss, possibly because it helps your body to break down fat more efficiently. Delicious, in many ways.

INGREDIENTS

* 60g **apricot jam**
* 1 tbsp fresh **ginger**, grated
* 450g lean **pork** tenderloin
* 1 tsp extra-virgin **olive oil**
* 280g frozen **okra**, chopped
* ½ **onion**, chopped
* 1 tsp dried **oregano**
* 250g frozen **corn kernels**
* 2 tsps **cider vinegar**
* 1 tsp **sugar**
* 3 tbsps thinly sliced **fresh basil**

METHOD

1/ Whack on your grill to get it ready for the pork. Then mix the jam and ginger in a bowl.
2/ Season the meat with a little salt and pepper. Grill for 10 minutes on each side. Brush with half of the jam mixture and cook for 2 minutes. Flip it over, brush with the rest of the mixture and cook another 2 minutes.
3/ For the succotash: heat the oil in a frying pan. Cook the okra, onion and oregano for 6 minutes. Stir in the corn, vinegar, sugar and basil, and cook until it starts to brown.
4/ Pop the meat on a chopping board, cover loosely with foil and let it rest 10 minutes. Then cut it into 16 slices. Mmm, smell that? Serve up with the succotash.

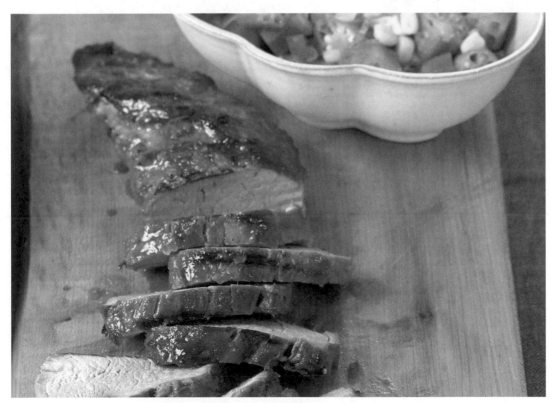

PHOTOGRAPHY: MIKI DUISTERHOF

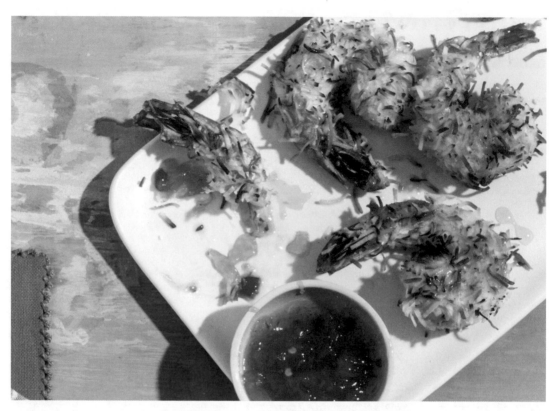

BAKED COCONUT PRAWNS

SERVES **4** | CALS **170** | SAT FAT **4.5g** | READY IN **20** MIN

WHY

Breaded prawns – it was the 1980s canapé of choice. Thirty years later, we're giving it a makeover by adding desiccated coconut. You'll get a satisfying 'bite' to your protein-full prawns and use less stodgy breadcrumbs, too. Oh and according to a study in *Physiology & Behavior*, cayenne pepper has been shown to curb your appetite and burn up to 10 per cent more calories for up to four hours after eating it. Wowza! Your tongue might not like it, but your waistline will.

INGREDIENTS

✱ 20 large **prawns**, peeled and de-veined
✱ 150g **panko breadcrumbs**
✱ 100g unsweetened **coconut flakes**
✱ Pinch **cayenne pepper**
✱ Pinch **chilli powder**
✱ 2 tbsps **flour**
✱ 1 **egg white**, beaten
✱ **Chilli sauce**
✱ **Lime** wedges

METHOD

1/ Roll up your sleeves and preheat your oven to 220°C. Line a baking sheet with foil and spray with olive-oil cooking spray.
2/ Rinse the prawns and set aside. In a plastic zip-lock bag, mix the breadcrumbs, coconut, cayenne pepper and chilli powder.
3/ Put the flour and egg white in separate small dishes. Dredge the prawns in the flour, dip into the egg, then gently shake them in the bag with the coconut mixture until coated.
4/ Place the prawns on the foil, lightly coat with cooking spray and bake for 12 minutes or until the coconut is browned. Serve warm with a squeeze of lime and a dollop of chilli sauce. Some like it hot, you know.

KICK-ASS QUINOA MEDLEY

 SERVES **2** CALS **742** SAT FAT **13g** READY IN **20** MIN

WHY

Not only does this salad look like a rainbow on your plate, it's also packed with enough easily digested protein to keep you from wanting to reach for the ice cream afterwards. Quinoa is low-GI and high-fibre so it'll stabilise blood-sugar levels. Plus, research in the journal *Obesity* suggests its phytonutrient content may even have anti-obesity properties.

INGREDIENTS

* ✱ ¼ **cucumber**, diced
* ✱ 1 **small head fennel**, cut thinly
* ✱ 50g **pomegranate seeds**
* ✱ 1 tbsp each chopped **flat-leaf parsley** and **mint**
* ✱ 50g sliced **radishes**
* ✱ 200g **cooked quinoa**
* ✱ 100g crumbled **feta cheese**
* ✱ 25ml **lemon juice**
* ✱ 1 tsp **pomegranate molasses**
* ✱ ½ tsp **sumac**
* ✱ 75ml **extra-virgin olive oil**

METHOD

1/ Prep all the salad ingredients and mix with the quinoa in a large bowl.
2/ Next, whip up the dressing by whisking the lemon juice, pomegranate molasses, sumac and olive oil together. Drizzle it over the vegetables and quinoa.
3/ Spoon it into bowls, top with feta and you're done. Who needs Pret?

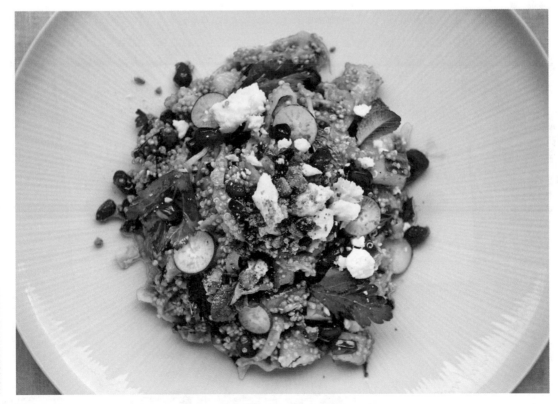

YOGI BARE CAFE

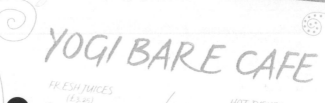

FRESH JUICES
(£3.25)

1 **Green Machine**
(Kale, celery, cucumber)

Very Cherry
(Cherry, mixed berries)

Top Banana
(Banana, pear, honey)

Beet Street
(Beetroot, apple, ginger)

PROTEIN SHAKES
(£3.95)

Hemp & Heavy
(Hemp protein, soy milk, mango)

Greek Goddess
(Whey protein, Greek yoghurt, berries)

Bees Knees
(Whey protein, banana, milk, honey)

SNACKS

Seedsation protein bars & balls £2

3 **Freshly popped corn £1.50**
Salt / Sweet / Sweet 'n' salt

Root vegetable crisps £1.25

HOT DISHES
(£9.50)

Organic Veggie burger

Vegetarian lasagne

Mung-bean casserole

Spicy tofu noodle stir-fry

Daily special
*(See the blackboard for
our seasonal specials)*

FRESH SALADS
(£6.50)

2 Leafy greens and seasonal local veg
topped with:
Chicken / Tofu / Halloumi

and a side of:
Quinoa / Lentils / Rice / Rye bread

(Dressed with balsamic vinaigrette)

DESSERTS

Raw chocolate sensation £4.50

4 **Vegan ice-cream £3**

Gluten-free cakes and bakes
(See the counter for our fresh selection)

THE *HEALTH* FOOD CAFE

Hey you, with your organic, gluten-free muffin and soya latte!
Careful: even the healthiest venues can be secret sugar silos

 ## DRINKS

CHOOSE:
Fresh juices. Avoid the pre-packaged kind, as pasteurisation damages antioxidants. And ditch high-GI juice ingredients (like banana or pineapple) for lower-GI fruits, like blueberries.

LOSE:
Only choose a protein shake if you've exercised in the past 30 minutes. Most have 100 calories a scoop, but it's the extras, like whole milk and yoghurt, that can take it nearer 450!

 ## SNACKS

CHOOSE:
Popcorn. It's 100 per cent unprocessed wholegrain, and most come in under 100 calories per bag. Plus, a recent study showed popcorn has more antioxidants than some vegetables.

LOSE:
Protein bars and balls. "They can pack in more than 200 calories," nutritionist Rose Chamberlain says. "Find ones with a sugar content lower than 15g per 100g," dietitian Sophie Claessens adds. Got that?

 ## MAINS

CHOOSE:
Pick a salad option with lean meat (chicken or turkey are best) and quinoa. Quinoa has seven times as much protein as brown rice, so it'll keep you full for longer.

LOSE:
"Avoid veggie burgers," says nutritionist Rose Chamberlain. Meat is bound with natural fats and can be grilled; veg burgers need to be deep-fried, which can up their calories by a huge 60 per cent.

 ## DESSERTS

CHOOSE:
Raw chocolate cake. It'll be calorie heavy (250 calories per slice) from the coconut oil, but your body converts its medium-chain triglycerides to energy rather than fat. Smart stuff.

LOSE:
Gluten-free goodies. "To make up for the lack of texture, most are loaded with sugar and fat," says nutritionist Danielle Collins. Gluten-free muffins can pack 20g fat and 450 calories. Forget it.

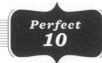

MAGIC-BITE SUSHI

If there's one kind of food that encourages mindful eating, it's the exquisite bite-sized treasures of sushi. Nourish your skin and body with these tiny, yet filling, works of art

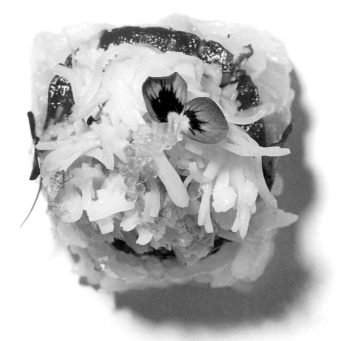

HUNGER-FIGHTING CRAB MAKI

Makes 6 pieces | Cals 115
20 mins

INGREDIENTS

* 40ml **rice vinegar**
* 20g **sugar**
* 10g **salt**
* 100g cooked **sushi rice**
* 20ml **mirin**
* 60g **mixed berries**
* 50g **crabmeat**
* 10g **spring onion**
* 40g **strawberries**
* 15g **sesame seeds**
* 5g **wasabi**

METHOD

To make the sushi rice: warm the vinegar, dissolve in the sugar and salt, mix in the rice and cool. Then warm 110ml water, 20ml rice vinegar and the mirin. Cool the rice, add the berries and blend. Chop the crabmeat, onion and strawberries. Cover the seaweed with rice and sprinkle with sesame seeds. Flip it over, add the chopped ingredients and roll. Garnish with wasabi. **Eastern promise:** Strawbs help to slow carb absorption, so you stave off hunger pangs. Happy days!

PHOTOGRAPHY: STUDIO 33 | RECIPES COURTESY OF CLAUDIO CARDOSO AND TAI PO WONG, EXECUTIVE CHEFS, SUSHISAMBA

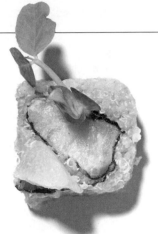

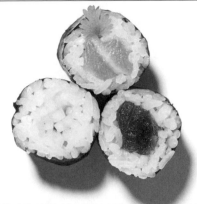

ANTI-AGEING YELLOWTAIL MAKI

Makes 6 pieces | Cals 80 | 15 mins

✹ 80g **quinoa** ✹ 1 piece **seaweed** ✹ 10g **caviar** ✹ 80g **yellowtail**
✹ 5g **chives**, chopped ✹ 60g **orange segments** ✹ 20g **coconut flakes**
✹ 20g **lemongrass** ✹ **Lime juice** ✹ 5g **wasabi**

Boil the quinoa for 10 minutes, cool and spread it over the
seaweed. Flip the seaweed and cover it with caviar. Add
yellowtail, chives, orange, coconut and chopped lemongrass.
Cut into pieces and garnish with lime juice and wasabi. **Eastern
promise:** Lemongrass has a mix of anti-ageing essential oils
that aid cell rejuvenation. Turn back the hands of time.

FLAT-BELLY SALMON HOSOMAKI

Makes 6 pieces | Cals 131 | 20 mins

✹ 40ml **rice vinegar** ✹ 20g **sugar** ✹ 10g **salt** ✹ 100g cooked
sushi rice ✹ 4 pieces **seaweed** ✹ 80g **cucumber** ✹ 70g **salmon**
✹ 100g **tuna** ✹ 20g **chives** ✹ 5g **wasabi**

Prepare the sushi rice as before. Next, spread the cooled
rice on to one sheet of the seaweed, add the chopped
cucumber and roll it up. Repeat for the salmon and tuna
sushi. Use chives and wasabi to garnish if desired. **Eastern
promise:** Tuna and salmon are filled with omega-3, great
for building lean muscle. The perfect post-gym snack.

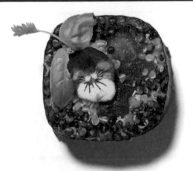

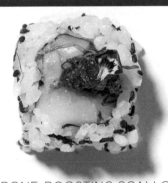

BRAIN-BUSTING TUNA MAKI

Makes 6 pieces | Cals 91 | 15 mins

✹ 80g **quinoa** ✹ 60g **red quinoa** ✹ 1 piece **seaweed**
✹ 70g **tuna** ✹ 70g **watermelon** ✹ 15g **basil**
✹ 20ml **light soy sauce** ✹ 5g **wasabi**

Boil both types of quinoa in a pan for 10 minutes, cover and
leave to cool. Lay out the seaweed and spread the quinoa in
the middle. Slice the tuna, place it over the quinoa with the
watermelon and basil, then roll it up! Garnish with soy sauce
and wasabi. **Eastern promise:** Seaweed is high in selenium,
which supports cognitive function. Eat yourself clever!

BONE-BOOSTING SCALLOP

Makes 6 pieces | Cals 152 | 25 mins

✹ 40ml **rice vinegar** ✹ 20g **sugar** ✹ 10g **salt** ✹ 100g cooked **sushi rice**
✹ 5g **rosemary** ✹ 25ml **honey** ✹ 10g **Dijon mustard** ✹ 70g **scallops**
✹ 25g **prunes** ✹ 10g **caviar** ✹ 1 piece **seaweed** ✹ 10g **black sesame
seeds** ✹ 15g **spinach** ✹ 15g **raisins** ✹ 5g **wasabi**

Prepare the rice, then chop the rosemary and mix with the
honey and mustard. Chop the scallops and prunes, add the
caviar and refrigerate. Spread the rice on the seaweed and
sprinkle with seeds. Flip and add the scallop mix, spinach
and raisins. Roll up, cut, serve with wasabi. **Eastern promise:**
Prunes protect against loss of bone density. Bone-us!

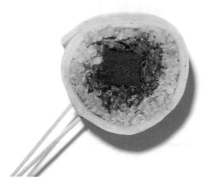

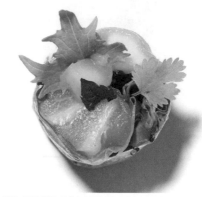

DETOXIFYING BEETROOT MAKI

Makes 6 pieces | Cals 52 | 4½ hours

✳ 80g **quinoa** ✳ 200g **cucumber** ✳ 70g **red onions** ✳ 30ml **beetroot juice** ✳ 15ml **rice vinegar** ✳ 25g **coriander**

Cook and cool the quinoa. Cut the cucumber into 14cm pieces, then peel off the skin, creating a long 'leaf'. Slice the onion, toss with the beetroot juice and vinegar and refrigerate for four hours. Fill the leaf with quinoa, coriander and the pickled onion. Roll, secure with skewers, then cut it up. **Eastern promise:** Beetroot helps to improve the liver's function to eliminate nasties. Win.

CARB-FREE SALMON AND GINGER MAKI

Makes 6 pieces | Cals 55 | 10 mins

✳ 100g **apple, peeled and chopped** ✳ 10g **ginger** ✳ 90g **mango, peeled and chopped** ✳ 10ml **rice vinegar** ✳ 1 piece **rice paper** ✳ 80g **rocket** ✳ 40g **tofu** ✳ 70g **salmon** ✳ **Coriander leaves**

Find your blender and zap the apple, ginger, 40g of the mango and vinegar to make a dressing, then strain. Next, wet the rice paper and add the rocket, the rest of the mango, tofu and salmon. Roll it up and cut into pieces. Serve with the dressing and coriander. **Eastern promise:** Top your sushi with anti-inflammatory ginger – nature's flat-belly antacid. Eat up!

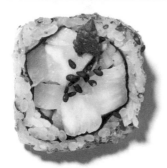

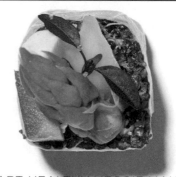

IMMUNE-BOOSTING MELON MAKI

Makes 6 pieces | Cals 92 | 20 mins

✳ 40ml **rice vinegar** ✳ 20g **sugar** ✳ 10g **salt** ✳ 100g cooked **sushi rice** ✳ 1 piece **seaweed** ✳ 5g **shichimi togarashi** ✳ 50g **melon** ✳ 50g **pineapple** ✳ 20g **cucumber** ✳ 10g **radish** ✳ 5g **wasabi**

You know the drill by now: prepare the sushi rice as before. Once it's cooked and has cooled down, sprinkle the seaweed with shichimi togarashi (a spice mix) and add your rice, melon, pineapple, cucumber and radish. Roll up, cut up, and dish up with wasabi. Done! **Eastern promise:** Pineapple is full of essential nutrients, enhancing the body's immune system. Sayonara, cold and flu season!

HEART-HEALTHY VEGGIE MAKI

Makes 6 pieces | Cals 79 | 20 mins

✳ 80g **quinoa** ✳ 1 **lettuce leaf** ✳ 50g **mango** ✳ 30g **avocado** ✳ 30g **cucumber** ✳ 35g **strawberries** ✳ 60g **passion fruit** ✳ 30g **asparagus** ✳ 50g **tofu** ✳ **Coriander** ✳ 5g **wasabi** ✳ 10g **pickled ginger**

Boil the quinoa in 110ml of water for 10 minutes. Let it cool, then spread it on to the lettuce leaf. Roll it up and cut into six pieces. Use the fruits, vegetables, tofu and coriander to uniquely garnish each piece. Serve with wasabi and pickled ginger. Veggie lovers, rejoice! **Eastern promise:** Tofu is made from soy beans, which help to lower blood pressure by reducing cholesterol in the blood. Stress relief in a bean.

LEAN SALMON ASPARAGUS MAKI

Makes 6 pieces | Cals 115
2½ hours

INGREDIENTS

* ✳ 40ml **rice vinegar**
* ✳ 20g **sugar**
* ✳ 10g **salt**
* ✳ 100g cooked **sushi rice**
* ✳ 350g **Granny Smith apples**
* ✳ 20ml **honey**
* ✳ 1 piece **seaweed**
* ✳ 80g **salmon**
* ✳ 60g **asparagus**
* ✳ 30g **tofu**

METHOD

Make the sushi rice as before. Heat 20ml water with 100g of the apples (peeled and chopped) and 5g of the honey to make a sauce. Cover the remaining thinly sliced apples with the rest of the honey and bake for two hours at 80°C. Spread the rice on the seaweed and flip it over. Add the salmon, asparagus, tofu and baked apples. Roll, cut into pieces, serve with apple slices and apple sauce. **Eastern promise:** Asparagus aids weight loss by detoxifying and cleansing the kidneys. They're slimming spears.

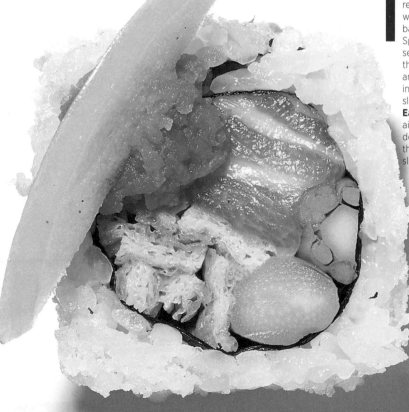

THAI
C U I S I N E

STARTERS

1 TOM YUM SOUP
£5.49

THAI CHICKEN SOUP
£4.00

THAI FISH CAKES
£4.99

CHICKEN SATAY
£5.95

DUCK SPRING ROLLS
£3.95

SUMMER ROLLS
£5.95

SPICY RIBS
£4.95

CURRIES

RED CURRY
£8.95

YELLOW CURRY
£10.95

GREEN CURRY
£6.95

JUNGLE CURRY
£9.99

FISH CURRY
£11.00

2 MASSAMAN
£8.95

KAENG PA
£9.95

PANANG CURRY
£12.00

DUCK CURRY
£7.50

NOODLES

PAD SEE EW
£8.95

PAD THAI
£9.95

PAD KEE MAO
£8.95

3 YUM WOON SEN
£6.95

RICE

COCONUT RICE
£1.99

KAO PAD FRIED RICE
£3.00

4 BROWN RICE
£2.00

JASMINE RICE
£1.95

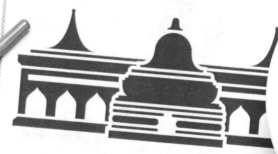

THE *THAI* RESTURANT

While strong flavours will kill sugar cravings, some high-calorie hazards are lying in wait for you. Here's how to avoid them

1 STARTERS

ORDER:
Fob off the fried stuff and have a broth-based tom yum soup. "Choosing tom yum over a satay gives you 12g less fat and about 500 fewer calories," says dietician David Tchilingirian. Soup spoon, ready?

AVOID:
Duck spring rolls and Thai fish cakes are some of the worst pickings on the menu. Both are deep-fried, packing at least 250 calories and 8g of fat per serving.

2 CURRIES

ORDER:
If you're craving a guilt-free curry, a kaeng pa is made with water rather than coconut milk and contains around 21g less saturated fat than other menu options.

AVOID:
When it comes to saturated fat, beef *massaman* is (sadly) the top offender, packing peanuts, cream, coconut milk, potatoes – and 680 calories per serving.

3 NOODLES

ORDER:
At 325 calories, a salad like yum woon sen is low in fat because the glass noodles aren't stir-fried. "Thai dressings tend to swap oil for chilli and lemon," says dietician Azmina Govindji. Perfect.

AVOID:
Pad Thai varies considerably in calories between restaurants. If you must, ask for it without the peanuts to cut 170 calories and 15g of fat. Nuts, eh?

4 RICE

ORDER:
Steamed jasmine rice is low in fat and has just 250 calories. But brown rice is the winner, packing twice as much fibre as rice noodles to keep you full.

AVOID:
Compared with steamed jasmine rice, *kao pad* fried rice adds a whopping 100 calories and 15g of fat. Go against the (fried) grain.

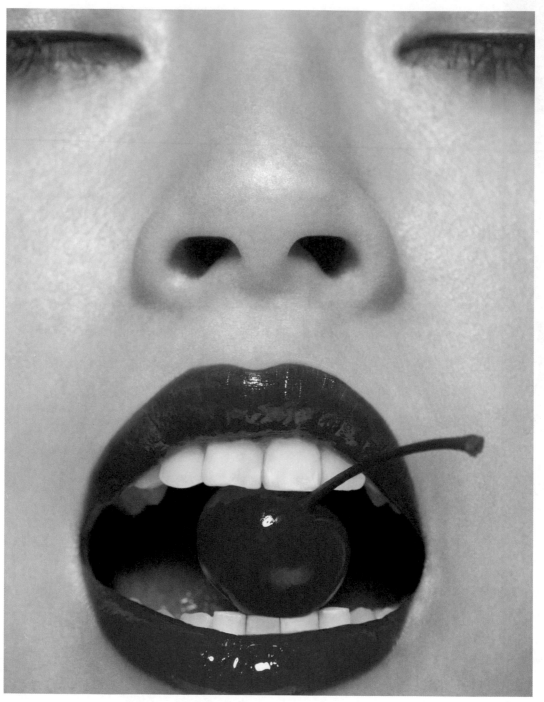

9

SWEET LIFE
TREATS

✦ DESSERTS ✦ BITES ✦ PUDDINGS ✦

You don't have to shun sweet treats forever to slim down your sugar belly – and did you know about the wealth of extra health goodies that raw desserts have to offer? The 20-day plan will have taught you how to minimise added sugar by making friends with fruit, but this chapter takes nature's greatest treat to the next level

208 Sweet Temptation
These delicious puddings and bakes harness the irresistible allure of natural fruit flavours, with minimal added sugar and a wealth of body-and-beauty-boosting antioxidants.

216 Speedy Treats
How quickly do you reach for a packet of sinful sugar snacks when cravings strike? Here are just a few tasty and quick-to-prepare alternatives to plump for... before you get plump.

218 Raw Desserts
Get ready to update your dessert skills with this impressive range of chocolatey, gooey, skin-boosting, energy-giving concoctions – none of which require any cooking!

SWEET TEMPT

MANGO COCONUT CHIA PUDDING

| SERVES 4 | CALS 280 | SAT FAT 6g | READY IN 70 MIN |

WHY

In our never-ending quest to find a sugar-free dessert that doesn't make us weep with disappointment, coconut milk is our latest ally. "Smooth, velvety textures are interpreted by the brain as sweet even when they aren't, so adding coconut milk to dishes and desserts will appease the dopamine receptors that crave sweetness at every turn," says Smith. No need to tell us twice.

INGREDIENTS

* 1 tin **light coconut milk**
* 40g **white chia seeds**
* 2 tbsps **honey**
* 1 tsp **vanilla extract**
* 1 **mango**, peeled, pitted and diced
* Handful **strawberries**, diced
* 30g sliced **almonds**
* 4 tsps **coconut flakes**

METHOD

1/ In a pint-size measuring cup, mix together the coconut milk, chia seeds, honey and vanilla. Stir until combined, then refrigerate for 1 hour.
2/ In four serving glasses, layer the pudding mixture and mango, then repeat three times. Top with strawberries, sliced almonds and a sprinkle of coconut. Ta da!

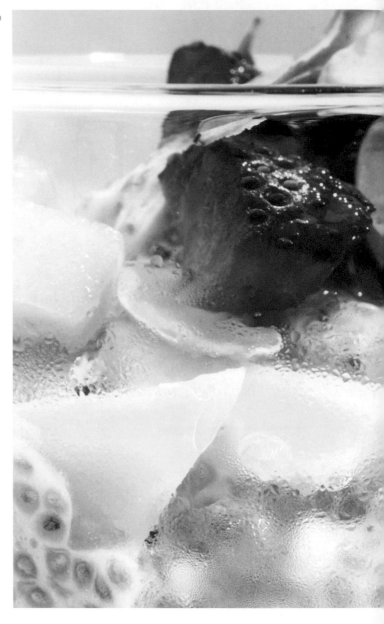

ATION

There's no room for 'make-do' substitiute puds here – grab a spoon and indulge, all the while sparing your waistline from harm

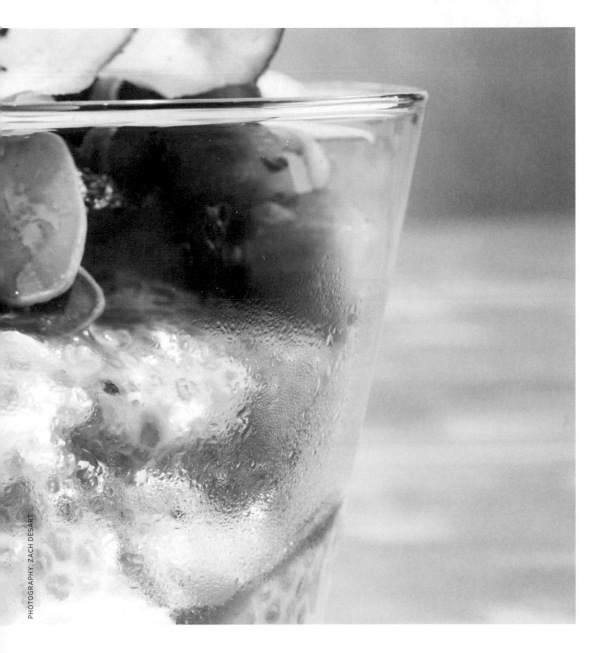

PHOTOGRAPHY: ZACH DESART

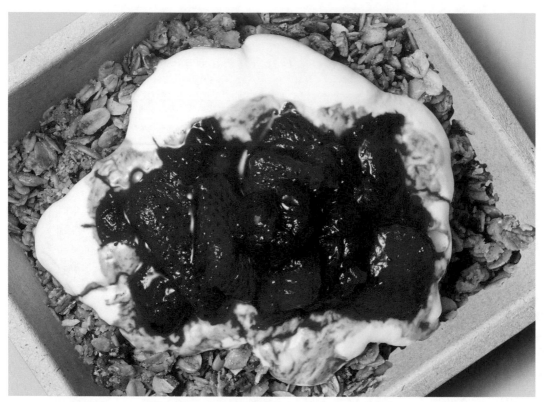

SUGAR-SMART SPICED CHERRY COMPÔTE

| SERVES 4 | CALS 76 | SAT FAT 00g | READY IN 20 MIN |

WHY

There's no need to reach for the jam jar when this compote is so easy to make – and just as delicious as its sugary cousin. Research shows cherries can reduce belly fat thanks to xylose, which is absorbed slowly and doesn't cause blood-sugar spikes. Sweet.

INGREDIENTS

* 250g **strawberries**, halved
* 250g **cherries**, stoned
* 2 **star anises**
* 1 stick **cinnamon**
* 1 tbsp **honey** or **agave syrup**
* **granola** (optional)

METHOD

1/ This one is so easy, you could do it with your eyes closed (probably best not to try it, though). Put all of the ingredients in a pan. Heat gently for 15 minutes until the strawberries and cherries have fully softened. Leave them to cool for a few minutes to allow the spices to infuse, then remove the star anises and cinnamon. This is delicious served on granola and will last for up to four days in the fridge (if it makes it that long).

PHOTOGRAPHY: STUDIO 33

METABOLISM-FIRING PINEAPPLE AND YOGHURT

 SERVES **2** — CALS **174** — SAT FAT **1.8g** — READY IN **12**MIN

WHY

If you hit the gym at lunch, this is one of the smartest snacks to keep in your recipe armoury. Bromelain in pineapple is great for helping digestion. Meanwhile, the chilli salt replenishes salt levels after your workout while revving your metabolism. Lastly, the protein in the yoghurt will not only help build up your muscles, it's also the number one satiety nutrient, stimulating the hormones that keep you full while cutting calorie intake. It's a shame Müller Crunch Corners don't count.

INGREDIENTS

* 200g diced **fresh pineapple**
* 1 tbsp torn **fresh mint leaves**
* 1 tsp **agave syrup**
* 200ml **Greek yoghurt**
* 1 tsp **chilli salt**

METHOD

1/ This is an easy one. Start by thinly dicing the pineapple, then add the mint and agave and mix well. Leave for 10 minutes to marinade and then serve with a dollop of the Greek yoghurt and a sprinkling of the chilli salt. That's it. No, really. That. Is. It.

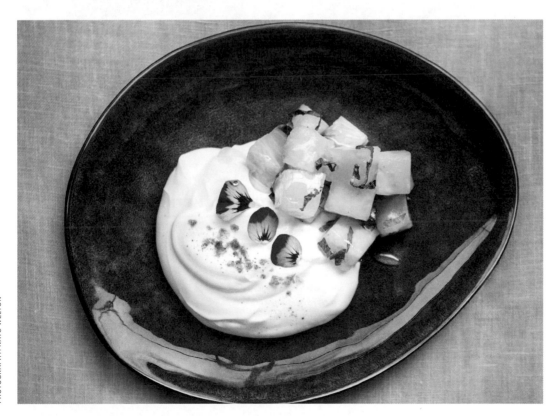

PHOTOGRAPHY: NATO WELTON

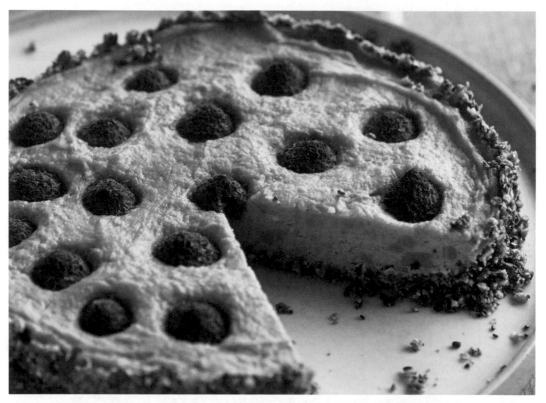

RASPBERRY-STUDDED BUTTERNUT SQUASH PIE

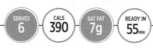

SERVES 6 | CALS 390 | SAT FAT 7g | READY IN 55 MIN

WHY

Squash is packed full of vitamins A, C, K and E, as well as magnesium, potassium and iron, which means it's excellent for hair volume, gloss and regrowth, as well as maintaining a healthy scalp. You can even use squash directly on your hair and scalp as an intensive conditioner. You heard us – get that pie on your head, pronto!

INGREDIENTS

* 105g raw **cashew nuts**
* 40g **sesame seeds**
* 1 ½ tbsps **chia seeds**
* 1 ½ tbsps **flaxseed**
* 40g **sunflower seeds**
* 60g cooked **brown rice**
* 60g **quinoa flakes**
* 6 drops **stevia liquid**
* 1 tsp **alcohol-free vanilla extract**
* ½ tsp **ground cinnamon**
* 2-3 tbsps **coconut oil** (and a little extra to grease the base)

METHOD

1/ It's pie time! Preheat your oven to 190°C and grease a 20cm cake tin or pie dish.
2/ Put the base ingredients in a processor, adding the coconut oil last; blitz for 15 secs.
3/ Remove the dough and, using your hands, press it evenly into the tin. Bake blind (with greaseproof paper on top covered in rice or baking beans) for 10-15 minutes.
4/ Now for the fun part: combine all the topping ingredients, except the raspberries, in a large bowl and mash with a fork until smooth. Spoon this mix into the base and stud with the raspberries. Return the pie to the oven and bake for 35 minutes. Serve warm or cold. Nigella, eat your heart out.

SWEET BAKED FIGS

SERVES 4 | **CALS** 270 | **SAT FAT** 2g | **READY IN** 15 MIN

WHY

For the dewiest skin imaginable, look no further than figs. Rich in complexion-boosting vitamin A, the figs in this healthy dessert come with a protein boost from the coconut yoghurt. You beauty.

INGREDIENTS

* 4 fresh **figs**
* Drizzle of **honey** or **agave syrup**
* 2 tbsp **coconut yoghurt**
* 1 tbsp **cunflower seeds**
* sprinkling **cacao nibs** (optional)

METHOD

1/ Wash the figs and remove their stalks. Score a cross in the tops of them and place in an ovenproof dish, crosses facing up. Drizzle with a little honey or agave.
2/ Roast at 180°C for around 10 minutes. Serve with yoghurt, a sprinkle of seeds and nibs.

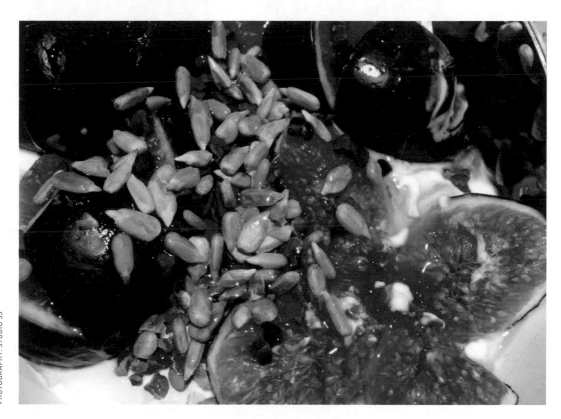

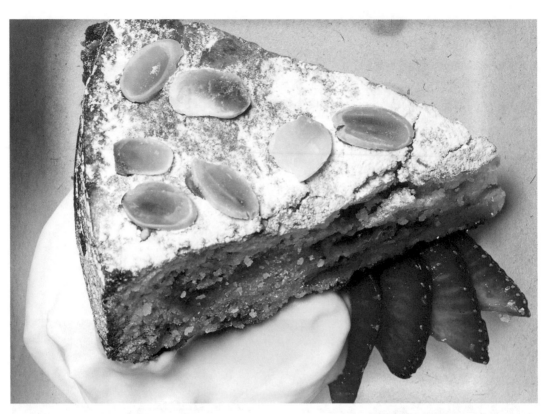

CRAVING-BUSTING ALMOND CAKE

PHOTOGRAPHY: STUDIO 33

SERVES	CALS	SAT FAT	READY IN
12	275	6g	75 MIN

WHY

WIth just 4 tsps of added sugar per serving, this cake takes most of its sweetness from the low-GI strawberries and almonds – which are packed with protein and fibre for slow-release energy. None of the usual cake-triggered blood-sugar meltdowns here; once you've enjoyed the last mouthful there won't be any craving-inducing dips half an hour afterwards.

INGREDIENTS

* 200g **self-raising flour**
* 1 tsp **baking powder**
* 50g **ground almonds**
* 200g **caster sugar**
* 350g **strawberries**
* 2 **eggs**
* 125g **plain yoghurt**
* 1 tsp **almond essence**
* 125g **butter**
* Handful **flaked almonds**, toasted

METHOD

1/ Start by preheating the oven to 180˚C. Next up: grease a 20cm spring-form cake tin and line it with parchment.

2/ Mix the flour, baking powder, almonds, sugar and a pinch of salt.

3/ Add the strawberries. Mix the eggs, yoghurt, almond essence and melted butter.

4/ Stir the wet mix into the dry mix until they're just combined. Bake for 50-60 minutes. Sprinkle on the flaked almonds.

PINEAPPLE, PISTACHIO & STRAWBERRY ICE CREAMS

SERVES 5

READY IN 60 MIN

WHY

All of these tempting ices are more like sorbets in their ingredients, but their skin, hair and nails-boosting nut content gives them a palate-pleasing creaminess to complement the antioxidant fruits.

METHOD

1/ This super-easy method works for all three. Whizz the ingredients in a blender, then churn the mix in an ice-cream maker until frozen. If you don't have one, freeze and pulse in a blender before serving with berries and biscotti. Cool.

PINEAPPLE

CALS 439

SAT FAT 6g

- ✳ 130g diced pineapple
- ✳ 250g macadamia nuts
- ✳ 1 tbsp grated ginger
- ✳ 5 tbsps agave nectar
- ✳ 130ml water
- ✳ Pinch sea salt

STRAWBERRY

CALS 231

SAT FAT 2g

- ✳ 130g fresh strawberries
- ✳ 130g cashew nuts
- ✳ 5 pitted medjool dates
- ✳ 1 tbsp agave nectar
- ✳ 130ml water
- ✳ Pinch sea salt

PISTACHIO

CALS 383

SAT FAT 2g

- ✳ 250g pistachio nuts
- ✳ 8 tbsps agave nectar
- ✳ Pinch cardamom
- ✳ 2 tbsps rose water
- ✳ 250ml water
- ✳ Pinch sea salt

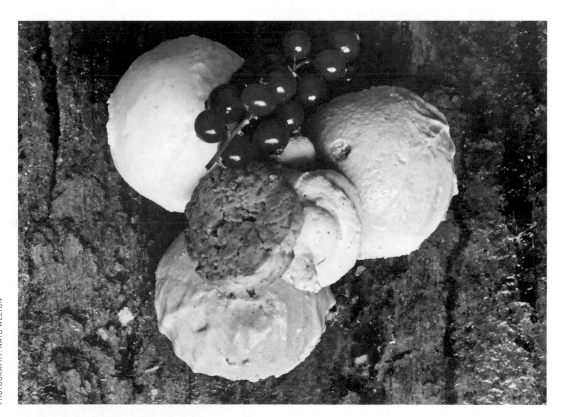

PHOTOGRAPHY: NATO WELTON

SPEEDY SNACK

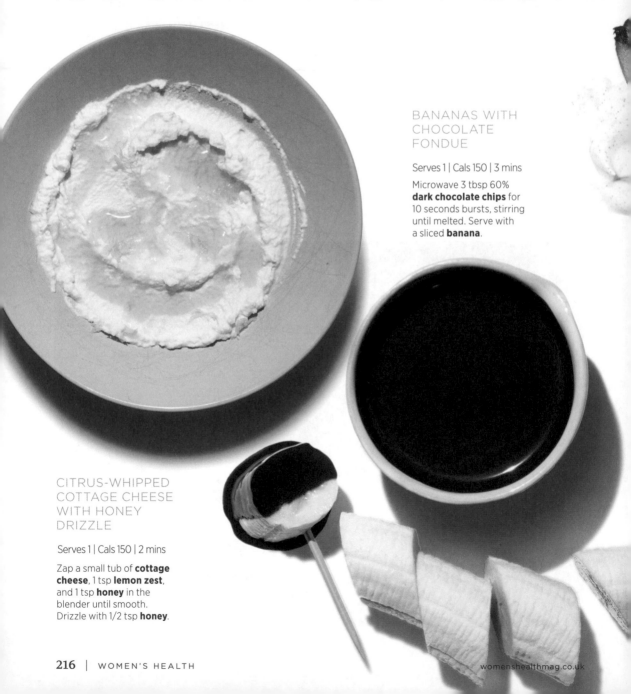

BANANAS WITH CHOCOLATE FONDUE

Serves 1 | Cals 150 | 3 mins

Microwave 3 tbsp 60% **dark chocolate chips** for 10 seconds bursts, stirring until melted. Serve with a sliced **banana**.

CITRUS-WHIPPED COTTAGE CHEESE WITH HONEY DRIZZLE

Serves 1 | Cals 150 | 2 mins

Zap a small tub of **cottage cheese**, 1 tsp **lemon zest**, and 1 tsp **honey** in the blender until smooth. Drizzle with 1/2 tsp **honey**.

SWAPS

Before you reach for something sugary to silence those cravings – stop! Here are just a few alternatives that are just as simple

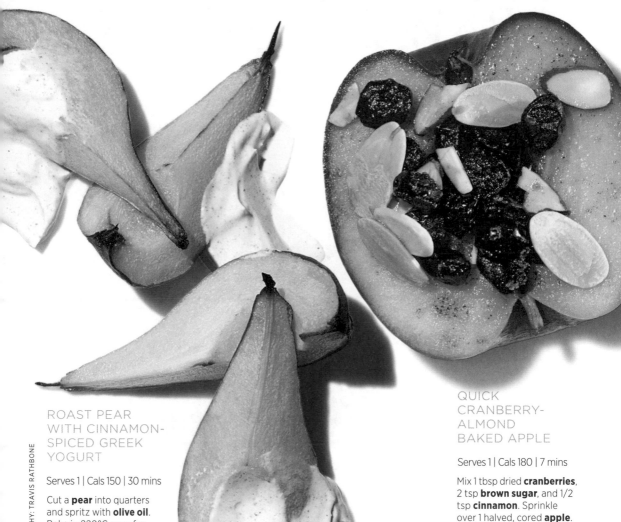

PHOTOGRAPHY: TRAVIS RATHBONE

ROAST PEAR WITH CINNAMON-SPICED GREEK YOGURT

Serves 1 | Cals 150 | 30 mins

Cut a **pear** into quarters and spritz with **olive oil**. Bake in 220°C oven for 20 minutes, until tender. Cool slightly, then top with 4 tbsp of **plain Greek yogurt** whisked with 1/2 tsp **agave nectar** and a big old pinch of **cinnamon**.

QUICK CRANBERRY-ALMOND BAKED APPLE

Serves 1 | Cals 180 | 7 mins

Mix 1 tbsp dried **cranberries**, 2 tsp **brown sugar**, and 1/2 tsp **cinnamon**. Sprinkle over 1 halved, cored **apple**. Cover and microwave until tender for 4 minutes. Cool slightly. Sprinkle with 1 tbsp sliced **almonds**.

RAW DESSERTS

*Sweet puds and treats with minimal added sugar that are actively good for you?
The dream. And also the reality when you delve into the realm of raw food*

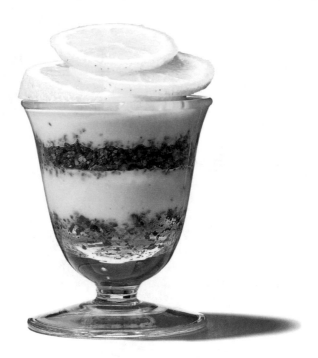

HOT-TROPIC
LEMON
CHEESECAKE

Serves 12 | 746 cals
35g sat fat | 80 mins'

INGREDIENTS

* 360g **pitted dates**
* 170g **walnuts**
* 115g **cacao nibs**
* 1½ tsp **vanilla powder**
* 450g **cashews,** soaked
* 100g **desiccated coconut**
* 330ml **coconut oil**
* Juice 9 **lemons**
* Zest 1½ **lemons**
* 15 drops **lemon essential oil**
* 110g **xylitol**
* ½ tsp **turmeric**

METHOD

Food processor still got juice? To make the biscuit layer, whizz the walnuts, cacao nibs and vanilla powder, then set aside. For the yummy-looking yellow 'cream', blend up all of the remaining ingredients. Line 12 glasses with cookie mix, pour a layer of cream until halfway and set it in the fridge for 1 hour. Repeat until the glass is full. **Cold comfort:** Dates are rich in potassium to help with digestion, anaemia and immunity. Win!

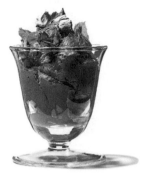

WHIP-ME CHOCOLATE MOUSSE

Serves 12 | 256 cals | 2g sat fat | 125 mins

✳ 6 **avocados** ✳ 480g **pitted dates,** soaked 4 hours ✳ 1½ tbsp **vanilla extract** ✳ 140g **cacao powder** ✳ ½ tsp **salt**

This one's so simple: all you have to do is put all of the ingredients in a blender and blend on high. Transfer into 12 small glasses, garnish with berries or dried flower petals and set in the fridge for 2 hours. Easy as. **Cold comfort:** One of the best natural forms of omega-9 fats, avocados help to lessen skin redness and irritation. Perfect.

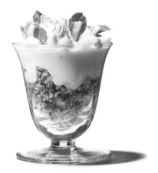

IF YOU LIKE PINA COLADA (CAKE)

Serves 12 | 450 cals | 16g sat fat | 130 mins

✳ **Base:** 175g **pitted dates** ✳ 320g **dried pineapple** ✳ 100g **desiccated coconut** ✳ 115g **almonds** ✳ 70g **macadamia** ✳ ½ tsp **salt** ✳ **Cream:** 225g **cashews**, skewed ✳ ½ **pineapple**, peeled ✳ 60ml **coconut nectar** ✳ 75ml **coconut oil** ✳ 10 drops **vanilla extract**

Soak the dates and dried pineapple for at least 1 hour (or they'll blow your mixer). Blitz the base items and line 12 glasses with equal amounts. For the cream, blend everything then fill glasses to the top. Garnish with macadamia and pineapple. **Cold comfort:** Not just for cheeky cocktails, pineapples are frothing with energy-boosting manganese.

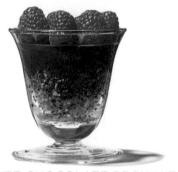

WOWEE CHOCOLATE BROWNIE

Serves 12 | 862 cals | 38g sat fat | 130 mins

✳ **Base:** 700g **pitted dates** ✳ 230g **walnuts** ✳ 230g **pecans** ✳ 120g **cacao powder** ✳ 2 tsp **sea salt** ✳ **Topping:** 480ml **coconut oil**, melted ✳ 120g cup **cacao powder** ✳ 4 tbsp **agave** ✳ 1 tsp **sea salt** ✳ handful **raspberries**

Blitz all the base bits until they form a sticky ball. Distribute evenly into 12 glasses. Stir topping items (sans raspberries) until smooth, pour over the brownie layer. Set it in the fridge for an hour, top with berries. Ta-da! **Cold comfort:** Being raw doesn't mean quitting chocolate. Cacao isn't processed, so it's rich in heart- and brain-boosting powers. Pew, pew!

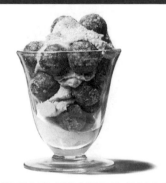

JINGLE ME (PROTEIN) BALLS

Serves 12 | 674 cals | 13g sat fat | 130 mins

✳ **Balls** (makes 60): 780g **pitted dates** ✳ 340g **almonds** ✳ 200g **hazelnuts** ✳ 170g **walnuts** ✳ 3 tbsp **tahini** ✳ 1½ tbsp **allspice** ✳ 1½ tbsp **cinnamon** ✳ 1½ tsp **sea salt** ✳ **Matcha cream:** 1½ **mango** ✳ 1½ tbsp **matcha powder** ✳ 3 tbsp **agave** ✳ 50g **desiccated coconut** ✳ 110ml **coconut oil**

Ball skills: process ingredients till they make a ball, roll into 120 tiny balls. Cream time: blend the peeled mango with the remaining items. Spoon into 12 glasses, sprinkle with 4 balls and repeat till glasses are full. Set in the fridge for 2 hours. **Cold comfort:** Green tea's clever cousin matcha is an antioxidant hub to help you ward off colds.

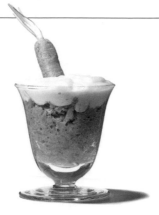

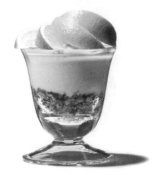

WHAT'S UP, DOC? CARROT CAKE
Serves 12 | 229 cals | 4g sat fat | 60 mins

✱ Cake: 160g **pitted dates**, soaked at room temperature ✱ 160g **dried apricots** ✱ 5 **carrots**, grated ✱ 115g ground **flaxseeds** ✱ 1 tbsp **cinnamon** ✱ 1 tsp **allspice** ✱ ½ tsp **sea salt** ✱ Icing: 150g **cashews**, soaked ✱ juice 1 **lemon** ✱ 3 tbsp **coconut oil** ✱ 3 tbsp **agave** ✱ 1 tsp **vanilla extract**

For the cake, pulse the fruit in a food processor until it's chutney-like. Add the remaining ingredients and process again. Distribute the mix into 12 glasses, leaving room at the top. For the icing, blend all the ingredients on high. Pour it over the cake. Dig in. **Cold comfort:** Carrots have beta-carotene to combat skin ageing – as beta-tested by Bugs.

TARTED-UP KEY LIME PIE
Serves 12 | 527 cals | 15g sat fat | 130 mins

✱ **Crust:** 380g **pitted dates** ✱ 120g **desiccated coconut** ✱ 50g **cacao powder** ✱ 140g **walnuts** ✱ 1 tsp **salt** ✱ Filling: ✱ 270g **lime juice** ✱ 360g **cashews**, soaked ✱ 1 **avocado** ✱ ½ **mango** ✱ 130ml **coconut butter** ✱ 90ml **agave**

Fancy some zest? Blitz all the crust ingredients then line 12 glasses with the mixture. Blend all the filling items until creamy and scoop into glasses. Relax while it sets in the fridge for 2 hours. (Wham! Christmas soundtrack optional.) **Cold comfort:** Cashews are rich in monounsaturated fats and have been shown to lower coronary heart disease risk. Nuts.

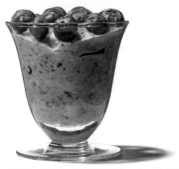

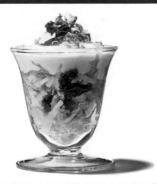

PURPLE RAIN BLUEBERRY PUDDING
Serves 12 | 345 cals | 14g sat fat | 130 mins

✱ Base: 140g **walnuts** ✱ 60g desiccated **coconut** ✱ 190g pitted **dates** ✱ 1 tsp **sea salt** ✱ Filling: 180g **cashews**, soaked ✱ 360g **blueberries** ✱ 130ml **coconut oil** ✱ 1 tbsp **stevia** ✱ 1 tbsp **vanilla powder** ✱ ⅓ tsp **sea salt**

The base is optional but if you're going for it, grind everything in a food processor and line the bottom of 12 glasses with mixture. Or go straight for the filling by blending everything on high and spooning into glasses. Garnish with blueberries. Let it set in the fridge for 2 hours. **Cold comfort:** The flavonoids in blueberries boost your memory – don't forget that.

WAHEY, IT'S MINCE PIE MADNESS
Serves 12 | 420 cals | 11g sat fat | 20+ mins

✱ **Filling:** 4 pears, **grated** ✱ 3 apples, **grated** ✱ 130g **raisins,** finely chopped ✱ juice 2 **oranges** ✱ zest 2 **oranges** ✱ 1½ tbsp **allspice** ✱ Frosting: 450g **cashews**, soaked ✱ 1 litre **coconut oil**, melted ✱ 1 litre **agave** ✱ juice 2 **lemons** ✱ zest 3 **oranges**

Combine all the filling gear in a bowl and let it marinate for 1-8 hours. Squeeze some juice out of the filling then distribute among 12 glasses. Blend the frosting ingredients on high, pour over the mince pie fillings and garnish with zest. **Cold comfort:** Allspice is a great source of vitamins A, B6 and C, plus an all-star gas reliever.

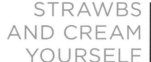

STRAWBS AND CREAM YOURSELF

Serves 12
338 cals | 17g sat fat
20 mins'

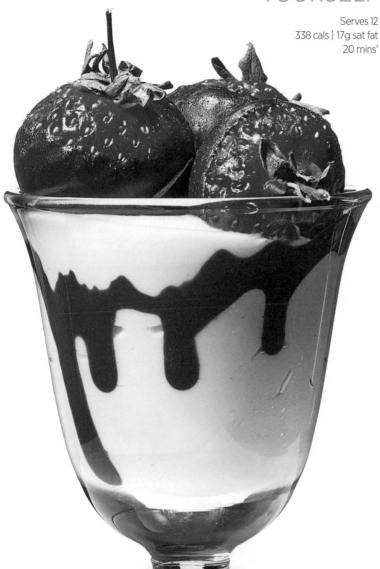

INGREDIENTS

✳ 36 **strawberries**, chilled

Chocolate sauce:
✳ 130g **cacao butter**, melted
✳ 75g **cacao powder**
✳ 2½ tbsp **agave**
✳ *Cream:* 360g **soaked cashews**
✳ 7 tbsp **coconut oil**
✳ 8 tbsp **agave**
✳ juice 2½ **lemons**
✳ 2½ tsp **vanilla extract**

METHOD

While your berries are chilling, stir all the sauce ingredients well. Dip strawberries in, holding the stalks and place on a non-stick tray to harden. Refrigerate. For the cream, blend all the bits, distribute among 12 glasses and top with 3 berries a glass. Keep in the fridge until serving. **Cold comfort:** Eat two servings of vitamin-C-filled strawberries and you're set for germ season. Boom.

PHOTOGRAPHY: STUDIO 33

RECIPE INDEX

INDEX

Women'sHealth

Editor **Edie Mullen**

Art Director **Graeme Sapsed**

Production **Roger Bilsland**

Sub Editors **Rachelle Harry, Lee Gale**

Picture Assistant **Arusha Mehta**

Editor-In-Chief **Farrah Storr**
Group Publishing Director
Alun Williams

Publisher **Duncan Chater**
Ad Manager **Chloe Barrington**
Senior Marketing Manager **Claire Matthews**

CEO, HEARST MAGAZINES UK
Anna Jones

HEARST-RODALE JOINT BOARD OF DIRECTORS
President and CEO, Hearst Magazines International
Duncan Edwards
Finance Director, Hearst Magazines UK
Jimmy Weir
Senior Vice President, Rodale International
Robert Novick
HEARST MAGAZINES UK
Director of Consumer Sales & Marketing **Reid Holland**
HR Director **Surinder Simmons**

Head of Newstrade Marketing **Jennifer Smith**
Circulation Manager **Bianca Lloyd-King**

RODALE INTERNATIONAL
Rodale Inc, 33 East Minor Street,
Emmaus, Pennsylvania 18098, USA
Editorial Director **John Ville**
Deputy Editorial Director **Veronika Taylor**
International Content Manager **Karl Rozemeyer**
Editorial Assistant **Natanya Spies**
Executive Director of Business Development
and Licensing **Kevin LaBonge**

Hearst-Rodale Ltd, 33 Broadwick Street, London, W1F 0DQ Tel: 020 7339 4400 Fax: 020 7339 4420